618.1\WHI

An Atlas of
THE MENOPAUSE

THE ENCYCLOPEDIA OF VISUAL MEDICINE SERIES

An Atlas of
THE MENOPAUSE

M.I. Whitehead, S.I.J. Whitcroft and T.C. Hillard

King's College Hospital
London, UK

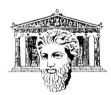

The Parthenon Publishing Group
International Publishers in Medicine, Science & Technology

Casterton Hall, Carnforth,
Lancs, LA6 2LA, UK

One Blue Hill Plaza, Pearl River,
New York 10965, USA

British Library Cataloguing-in-Publication Data
Whitehead, Malcolm I.
  Atlas of the Menopause. – (Encyclopedia of Visual Medicine
series)
  I. Title II. Series
  612.665
  ISBN 1-85070-388-4

Library of Congress Cataloging-in-Publication Data
Whitehead, Malcolm I.
  An atlas of the menopause/ M. I. Whitehead, S. I. J. Whitcroft
and T. C. Hillard
      p.   cm. – (The Encyclopedia of visual medicine series)
  Includes bibliographical references and index.
  ISBN 1-85070-388-4: $70
  1. Menopause–Complications–Diagnosis–Atlases. 2.
Menopause–Hormone therapy–Atlases. I. Whitcroft, S. I. J.
II. Hillard, T. C. III. Title. IV. Series.
  [DNLM: I. Menopause–atlases. WP 17 W592a 1993]

RG 186. W47 1993
618.1'75–dc20
DNLM/DLC
for Library of Congress   93-22687
                                                    CIP

Published in the UK and Europe by
The Parthenon Publishing Group Limited
Casterton Hall, Carnforth
Lancs. LA6 2LA

Published in North America by
The Parthenon Publishing Group Inc.
One Blue Hill Plaza
PO Box 1564, Pearl River
New York 10965, USA

Copyright © 1993 Parthenon Publishing Group Ltd

First published 1993

Typeset by AMA Graphics Ltd., Preston
Printed and bound in Spain by T.G. Hostench, S.A.

Contents

The Encyclopedia of Visual Medicine Series

Titles currently planned in this series include:

An Atlas of Oncology

An Atlas of Hypertension

An Atlas of Common Diseases

An Atlas of Osteoporosis

An Atlas of Contraception

An Atlas of Endometriosis

An Atlas of Ultrasonography in Obstetrics and Gynecology

An Atlas of Practical Radiology

An Atlas of Psoriasis

An Atlas of Trauma Management

An Atlas of Lung Infections

An Atlas of Transvaginal Color Doppler

An Atlas of Child Health

An Atlas of Infective Endocarditis

An Atlas of Rheumatology

An Atlas of Epilepsy

An Atlas of HIV and AIDS-related Diseases

An Atlas of Practical Dermatology

An Atlas of Laser Operative Laparoscopy and Hysteroscopy

An Atlas of Atherosclerosis

An Atlas of Eye Diseases

An Atlas of Cutaneous Growths

An Atlas of Myocardial Infarction

Series Foreword

The art of effective diagnosis is one that relies to a considerable degree – although certainly not exclusively – on the recognition of visual signs and manifestations of disease. The objective of the Series is to provide a practical aid to diagnosis by illustrating and explaining the wide range of visual signs that a physician needs to be aware of in current medical practice.

Whilst the visual manifestations of disease themselves remain constant, the development of new techniques of invasive and non-invasive diagnosis mean that new images are frequently being added to the range of visual material that the diagnostician must be familiar with: ultrasound, radiology, magnetic resonance imaging, endoscopy and photomicrography all provide examples of this kind of material. It is the intention of this Series to document, where appropriate, the result of such techniques and to explain and elucidate their relevance – in addition to documenting all the more standard visual images.

The Series is also distinctive in that individual volumes will focus on carefully selected, specific topics, which can be covered in some detail – rather than on generalized and broadly-based subject areas that could not easily be covered so thoroughly.

The authors contributing to the Series have all been selected for their special expertise in their own chosen fields, their access to outstanding visual material and their ability to explain the significance of it in an effective and lucid way. Finally, particular emphasis is being placed on achieving a very high quality of colour reproduction in the printing process itself in order to do full justice to the wide variety of visual images presented.

It is hoped that this carefully structured and systematic approach to the visually significant aspects of medicine will make a valuable and ongoing contribution to good diagnostic practice.

Introduction

The menopause is associated with symptoms of estrogen deficiency which may be extremely debilitating and seriously reduce the quality of life. Additionally, the increased risk of cardiovascular disease and osteoporosis, which occur with loss of ovarian function, has important implications for a modern society which is looking to prevent these avoidable conditions in an aging population.

Although it is well known that the menopause may occur in women who are in their teens and early twenties and may also be delayed until the late fifties, the average age at the menopause in the United Kingdom remains at 51 years, and overall this has not changed since records began. As female life expectancy increases to greater than 80 years, many women will now spend almost 40% of their lives in the postmenopausal state. As a result of this increased longevity, postmenopausal women now comprise approximately 17% of the population of the United Kingdom and this proportion can be expected to rise as family size in the Western world shrinks whilst life expectancy increases. Clearly, therefore, it is extremely important to safeguard the health of this generation in order to avoid a huge burden on society in future years.

The number of oocytes diminishes steadily throughout the female lifetime, and by the perimenopausal years those remaining respond poorly to stimulation by pituitary gonadotropins. With increasing age, structures within the ovary alter. The numbers of theca interna cells and granulosa cells – sites of production of progestogens and estrogens – are reduced, whilst interstitial cells increase, these being sites of androgen production.

Although the actual cessation of menses is an important milestone, the estradiol levels will gradually fall in the years immediately prior to the menopause as the number of oocytes reduces. This time is marked by a rise in the levels of gonadotropin follicle stimulating hormone (FSH) and luteinizing hormone (LH). Symptoms of estrogen deficiency can, therefore, occur several years before menstruation actually ceases and, during this time, levels of sex hormones can fluctuate. During this perimenopausal phase, increasing ovarian unresponsiveness leads to sporadic ovulation.

These anovulatory cycles are characterized by low estradiol levels and absence of a progesterone surge due to absent corpus luteum function. Menses may become irregular. Eventually, estradiol levels fall so low that endometrial proliferation no longer occurs and menstrual periods cease.

After the ovaries have ceased to function, the production of estrogen, by conversion from androstenedione, continues in small and variable amounts in extra-ovarian sites such as body fat and muscle, as well as from the adrenal glands. This peripheral conversion explains the relatively high level of estrogen seen in obese postmenopausal women and may also explain the higher than average risk of endometrial carcinoma in these women. Additionally, the postmenopausal ovary may also account for some estrogen production, although the relative amount is unclear.

During the premenopausal years, the predominant estrogen is estradiol, whereas the estrogen produced from the peripheral conversion in the postmenopausal years is the less biologically active estrone. Therefore, the estradiol to estrone ratio appears to be reversed after the menopause. The decline in estrogen production leads to a relative excess of androgens in the postmenopause, giving rise to androgenic features such as greasy skin, acne and facial hair as well as adverse changes in lipid profiles, which may influence the long-term risk of cardiovascular disease.

Section 1 A Review of the Menopause

Consequences of estrogen deficiency

In the female, lack of estrogens can affect many different tissues, and symptoms may, therefore, be of many different types, the severity varying between individuals. Symptoms may be acute, such as those of vasomotor instability, including hot flushes and night sweats. Conversely, their onset may be slower and more gradual due to the longer-term deprivation of estrogen, such as in urogenital atrophy.

Vasomotor instability

The most well-recognized symptom of the menopause is the hot flush. Visible signs are reddening of the skin, due to peripheral vasodilatation, accompanied by profuse sweating. The beginning of the flush appears to be marked by an increase in vascular perfusion to the periphery[1], with an associated increase in peripheral temperature. This is followed by an increase in serum LH, and subsequently a drop in core temperature, during which time the woman may complain of feeling cold and also experience palpitations, dizziness, nausea and panic attacks.

These flushes and associated symptoms may occur infrequently, or may occur so often, both day and night, that they significantly affect the patient's lifestyle. They may occur spontaneously or may be provoked by factors such as alcohol, stress and hot weather. They tend to be more severe in women who have undergone sudden and early loss of ovarian function, such as after bilateral oophorectomy or radiotherapy, and it is thought that a gradual decline in estradiol levels may allow a relative adjustment to the low estrogen levels.

Although it is estimated that around 75% of post-menopausal women will experience hot flushes and night sweats, in the majority the frequency and severity of these will diminish with time, eventually disappearing. In approximately 5% of women, however, these symptoms will continue indefinitely. Night sweats may cause night wakening and poor sleep patterns in many postmenopausal women, eventually leading to chronic tiredness and irritability.

It has been shown that in women describing night wakening, vasomotor flushes occurred at the time of the wakening episodes and there was a reduction in the duration of the important rapid eye movement (REM) sleep[2]. Partial wakening was, therefore, occurring on a much greater scale than was recognized by the patient.

Psychological symptoms

The number of women who suffer symptoms of depression, anxiety, forgetfulness and panic attacks increases at or around the menopause, and, despite the paucity of well-designed studies on this subject, most clinicians now accept that there is an endocrine component in many women so troubled.

Certainly, the increase in psychological symptoms seen in association with hot flushes and night sweats[3], and their previously described interference with normal sleep patterns, suggests that this may lead to chronic fatigue, depressed mood and inability to cope.

Nevertheless, this is a difficult subject to evaluate objectively, as it embodies interactions between all the events which may occur around this time of life, including illness and death of parents, divorce, problems with children and, finally, depression over children leaving home – the so-called 'empty-nest syndrome'. Furthermore, it has been shown that, as with menorrhagia, perception of the event of the menopause can have a profound effect on a woman's response to loss of ovarian function. For example, some women see the end of menstrual bleeds as a welcome release from an inconvenience and will welcome the menopause. As a result, they may suffer less than a woman who may have been preconditioned to expect an unpleasant time, perhaps because their mother had suffered more severely than usual during the menopause.

Position in society may also have a role to play. In many, especially non-western, societies the menopause will afford the woman status and privileges which may make her view this time as one to which to look forward in a positive way. The attitude of the developed world is, however, very different, favoring youth, and frequently neglecting older people. Not surprisingly, the occurrence of the menopause will only serve to underline the advancement of age, a view which may well be reinforced by the onset of symptoms of estrogen deficiency.

Additionally, with an increasing number of women remaining in employment well into their fifties and beyond, there is understandably less tolerance of the symptoms which their mothers often suffered without complaint. With an increasing tendency to discuss a subject which was once taboo, and with higher expectations for quality of life, a more informed population is increasingly inclined to opt for treatment rather than to suffer in silence.

Which group of women are genuinely suffering from endocrine-related psychological symptoms is, therefore, often difficult to establish. The importance of a good history cannot be emphasized enough, especially when other classical physical symptoms of estrogen deficiency do not accompany the psychological ones. It is important to question timing of onset of symptoms and to establish also whether similar symptoms occurred at other times associated with low estrogen levels, such as during the postnatal period.

Clearly, although it is undesirable to overlook a true endogenous depression and to attribute symptoms solely to the menopause, in some cases where diagnosis is difficult a trial of hormone replacement therapy may be beneficial; a trial is preferable and may be less potentially damaging than embarkation upon treatment with antidepressants straight away. An initial treatment period with estrogens for approximately 3 months, if successful, will differentiate between estrogen deficiency causing depressed mood and psychiatric depression. This time period is long enough to show a greater effect than would be attributable to placebo.

Connective tissue

Estrogen and androgen receptors have been identified on fibroblasts in the skin[4]. Skin is mainly made up of collagen fibers, the remainder being elastin. The dermis also contains a capillary network of veins, lymphatic channels, sebaceous glands and hair follicles. Sex steroids appear to have a direct effect on connective tissue, with estrogens increasing the intracellular fluid content, whilst testosterone causes proliferation of fibroblasts. Estrogen deficiency can lead to a reduction in collagen formation in connective tissues, including skin. This results in a decrease in skin thickness; treatment with estrogen or estrogen and testosterone appears to reverse these changes[5]. Other collagen effects commonly described around the menopause are an increase in joint pains, dry hair, brittle nails, sore eyes and gum shrinkage; these may respond to hormone replacement therapy to a variable extent.

Urogenital tissue

The urethra and vagina both contain estrogen receptors and are sensitive to changes in systemic concentrations of estrogen. Falling estradiol levels after the menopause lead to reduced vascularity of the tissue, along with a decrease in the glycogen content of the cells, which in turn leads to a fall in lactobacilli content and an increase in pH. This encourages the growth of certain bacteria including coliforms and streptococci.

Vaginal tissue contains three layers of cells. The parabasal cells lie above the basement membrane. Above these are the intermediate cells, and above these are the superficial cells. With a decrease in estrogen, more parabasal and fewer superficial cells are seen and these changes are reversed with estrogen replacement.

Atrophic changes produce symptoms of vaginal dryness, soreness and dyspareunia; replacement of estrogen, even in small amounts, is effective in reversing vaginal atrophy and increasing vaginal lubrication.

Miscellaneous

Other symptoms associated with the menopause exist but may not come into any strict category. Nevertheless, some are associated with a fall in estradiol levels and respond to a correction of these levels. These may include breast tenderness, abdominal bloating, paresthesiae, leg cramps and worsening headaches which may even become migrainous. Although the etiology of these symptoms is unclear, some may be attributable in part to an increase in fluid retention which can occur in the postmenopause. Many of these symptoms can occur to a varying extent with both estrogen deficiency, and as a side-effect of estrogen treatment, particularly with overdosage.

Long-term consequences of the menopause

Osteoporosis

The rate of bone loss increases in the years immediately following the menopause. This is mainly due to a disturbance in the balance between resorption and formation, with an overall increase in resorption. Although there is a gradual age-related decline in bone density, the most important factor in post-menopausal osteoporosis is loss of estrogen. Postmenopausal bone loss particularly affects the distal radius, the neck of the femur and the vertebral bodies. This leads to an increase in fracture at these sites, classically with minimal trauma.

Fracture of the hip is a condition associated with great pain and disability; osteoporosis of the spine leads to crush fractures of the vertebral bodies, eventually presenting as the Dowager's hump with severe kyphosis and respiratory and cardiovascular embarrassment.

It is estimated that, by the end of the seventh decade, 50% of women in the UK will have experienced an osteoporotic fracture[6]. The associated mortality and morbidity are very high; 20% will die as a direct result of hip fracture and approximately 50% will never regain full independence[7]. Furthermore, apart from the pronounced distress caused by this condition, approximately £700 million is spent annually as a direct consequence of osteoporosis. Clearly, prevention of osteoporosis pays dividends in the long term. As the postmenopausal female population increases towards 10 million, this problem is well worth addressing.

Low bone density is associated with small, slim, Caucasian women. A family history of osteoporosis[8], a sedentary lifestyle, increased alcohol and nicotine consumption, as well as long episodes of amenorrhea, will also increase the risk of osteoporosis. The risk of a woman experiencing an osteoporotic fracture within her lifetime depends upon two factors: the peak bone mass achieved and the rate of bone loss after the menopause. As the peak bone mass is largely genetically determined, it is difficult to influence; therefore, attempts to reduce the risk of subsequent fracture rest mainly with prevention of bone loss. Once bone mass is lost, attempts to reverse this process are limited, and therefore prevention by early diagnosis and prophylactic therapy is extremely important.

Loss of bone may occur in the perimenopause, particularly from the hip, as estradiol levels start to decline[9]. After the menopause, however, bone loss accelerates and between 3 and 5% of bone density may be lost annually for the first 5 years after menopause. Therefore, those women who have relatively low bone density at the beginning of the climacteric may be at greatly increased risk of fracture by age 55–60 years.

Although the maximum bone loss occurs in the first 5 years after the menopause, a reduction in bone density continues after this time. As life expectancy increases, prevention of further loss is clearly worthwhile, even in women over the age of 60.

Clearly, with an increasing proportion of the population being affected by this condition, it may be argued that there is a place for offering preventative treatment to all women. However, not all women are able or willing to take preventative steps and therefore screening remains an important factor in distinguishing those at high risk. Dual photon absorptiometry (DPA) and dual energy X-ray absorptiometry (DEXA) are the only reliable methods of measuring bone density in the spine and hip; the latter method will also measure total body bone density. These are becoming increasingly available, and are being evaluated for use in routine screening of the whole population.

Cardiovascular disease

Despite a tendency to consider cardiovascular disease as being primarily of male importance, arterial disease is the leading cause of death in postmenopausal women in Western countries.

It has been shown that premature menopause conveys a relatively high risk of developing coronary heart disease[10,11] and stroke[12], whilst postmenopausal estrogen replacement therapy reduces the risk of coronary heart disease[13,14] and stroke[12], by over 50%. Although the precise mechanism is still unclear, this may be due in part to the effect on lipid profiles. Loss of ovarian function leads to an increase in total and low density lipoprotein (LDL)-cholesterol, and a reduction in high density lipoprotein (HDL)-cholesterol particularly the HDL_2 subfraction. These changes are associated with an increased incidence of cardiovascular disease, and appear to be partially reversed in women taking estrogen replacement[15].

More recently, estradiol receptors have been demonstrated in the muscularis of premenopausal arteries[16], and preliminary studies using Doppler measurements of resistance to blood flow have suggested that loss of endogenous estradiol leads to an increase in resistance to blood flow in the uterine arteries[17] and, most recently, the carotid arteries[18]. This direct effect of estrogen on the vasculature may account for a great proportion of the changes in cardiovascular disease risk seen in the postmenopause.

Other factors in the cardiovascular equation are being increasingly investigated, including the impact of estrogen and progesterone on coagulation and carbohydrate metabolism; these are important areas for future research as are the effects of estrogens and progestogens on the vascular endothelium.

Benefits of hormone replacement therapy

Many placebo-controlled studies have shown that hormone replacement therapy relieves hot flushes and sweats; the improvement may be almost immediate or more gradual.

In a double-blind placebo-controlled cross-over study of 64 postmenopausal women with severe symptoms of estrogen deficiency including flushes, sweats and psychological symptoms[19], there was a significant reduction in the latter with use of estrogens as compared to placebo. However, an analysis of the results showed that many psychological symptoms were reduced only in women who had complained of vasomotor symptoms at the beginning of the study. This suggested that estrogens indirectly influence psychological status. However, poor memory was improved by estrogens independent of relief of hot flushes. Estradiol receptors have been identified in brain tissue. Schiff and co-workers found that the use of oral conjugated equine estrogens 0.625 mg daily significantly improved sleep patterns when compared to placebo[20]. It is increasingly believed that chronic interruption of sleep may contribute to many of the psychological symptoms of the menopause.

Urogenital symptoms

There is no doubt that treatment with estrogen relieves the classical symptoms of vaginal dryness and soreness associated with the menopause, and this may be achieved with both systemic and topical estrogens. Occasionally, women suffering only from urogenital symptoms may opt to use topical estrogens

only. This is particularly appropriate in those who are at low risk from the long-term consequences of the menopause and who do not wish to take systemic estrogens, whether because of a wish to avoid bleeds or because of a natural disinclination or for any other reason. There is concern, however, that those who use topical estrogens frequently and at high dose may put themselves at risk of systemic absorption. This is clearly undesirable when the uterus is intact and requires progestogen addition.

As well as reducing vaginal dryness and dyspareunia, estrogen replacement therapy has been shown in some studies to improve sexual interest and satisfaction, lack of which is cited as a cause for concern in women aiming to maintain marital harmony. The success of estrogen therapy in this respect may also be due to the general increase in well-being associated with replacement of estrogen. Some women find that estrogen replacement itself is not adequate to improve sexual interest, and occasionally treatment with small doses of testosterone may help. This appears to be particularly relevant in young women who have undergone surgical loss of ovarian function, and these women often require higher estrogen doses.

The bladder and associated structures also respond to treatment with estrogen. Estrogen administration increases the vascularity of estrogen-dependent tissues and, as in vaginal epithelium, its use leads to an increase in the number of superficial cells in the urethral epithelium as well as transitional cells in the elastic tissue in the urethra. The urethral syndrome describes the triad of urinary frequency, urgency and nocturia which may follow menopause, and these symptoms may be relieved with estrogen replacement. Stress incontinence may worsen around the menopause, but interestingly does not appear to be so responsive to treatment with estrogen as other urinary symptoms[21].

Clearly, there are many symptoms which may be attributable to the menopause, especially since estradiol receptors are found in so many tissues throughout the female. There is no doubt that many women achieve significant relief from these symptoms with hormone replacement therapy. It has been shown that, after instigating treatment, maximum symptom relief is often not seen until the end of the third treatment cycle[22]. It is important to allow a sufficient interval after treatment has been started before attempting to assess the efficacy of therapy. This should be stressed to patients who may have been misled by wild and enthusiastic claims from the lay press and other users of hormone replacement therapy, so as to avoid an unrealistic expectation of sudden and dramatic improvement in all symptoms.

In those who wish to withdraw from treatment for any reason, it is always wise to advise a gradual reduction in dosage of estrogen, as sudden withdrawal of treatment may lead to a recurrence of symptoms such as hot flushes.

Osteoporosis

At present, estrogen replacement therapy is the most widely used treatment given to reduce the rate of postmenopausal bone loss[23,24]. Estrogens are now normally given continuously without a 7-day break. The doses are given in Table 1.

Treatment should commence at or around the menopause and the longer the duration of treatment the greater the benefit in prevention of fractures in the long term. It has been calculated that 5 years of estrogen therapy started soon after the menopause will halve the fracture incidence[25]. There are, however, women who cannot or who are unwilling to take hormone replacement therapy. There is, therefore, a place for non-estrogen drug therapy. Newer agents include calcitonin, which directly inhibits bone

resorption. This may be used both for the prevention of osteoporosis[26] and for the treatment of established osteoporosis[27].

Bisphosphonates, which are analogues of pyrophosphate, and whose use has been established in the treatment of Paget's disease and malignancy-induced hypercalcemia, have shown promise in the prevention of postmenopausal bone loss[28]. These also reduce osteoclast activity but are given cyclically because they are retained within bone far longer than estrogens or the calcitonins. This ensures that bisphosphonates do not result in old bone being preserved at the expense of new.

There has been much debate as to the importance of calcium supplementation of the diet in preventing bone loss. Although some studies have shown that bone density may be slightly increased by calcium, nevertheless, the majority of epidemiological and histological studies have refuted this. There may, however, be a place for calcium supplements in those women whose diet would otherwise provide less than the statutory 400 mg daily requirement.

The effect of exercise in preventing bone loss remains under question. It does appear that regular weight-bearing exercise can produce a modest beneficial effect on bone density in the hip, although this is not as marked as that seen with estrogen therapy. However, it clearly has a place either on its own or in conjunction with estrogen therapy; and its advantages in maintaining general health, mobility and muscle strength should not be underestimated. These factors are all important, not only in reducing fracture risk by decreasing the likelihood of falls, but in preserving quality of life overall.

However, in pre- or perimenopausal women who are not receiving exogenous estrogens, excessive exercise can lead to hypothalamic disturbance, anovulation and a resulting fall in sex steroid production, which can adversely affect bone density.

Table 1 Bone conserving doses of estrogen

Conjugated equine estrogens	0.625 mg daily
Oral estradiol valerate	2 mg daily
Estradiol (transdermal)	50 μg daily
Estradiol implant	50 mg

Prevention of bone loss currently relies upon estrogens or calcitonin or a bisphosphonate restoring the balance between bone formation and resorption. Although stimulants of new bone formation, such as anabolic steroids and fluoride, have been studied, they can cause significant side-effects, at least at the doses so far examined. Therefore, until further data are available confirming safety, we believe that these stimulants do not warrant a place in the routine prevention of osteoporosis.

Cardiovascular disease

Although, up until the last two decades, the majority of studies on the patterns of cardiovascular disease were mainly in men, more recently a greater emphasis has been placed upon the large number of women affected by this disease. Use of oral estrogen therapy reduces total and low density lipoprotein (LDL)-cholesterol levels and increases high density lipoprotein (HDL)-cholesterol levels, but also increases plasma triglyceride levels[15]. The first studies which looked at the impact of estrogen on lipids and lipoproteins concentrated on the use of oral conjugated equine estrogens; however, there is now much more interest in different types of estrogen, the route of administration and the effects on lipid profiles. More recently, it has been shown that use of transdermal estrogen is as beneficial as oral estrogen in reducing total and LDL-cholesterol but yet does not have the same potentially adverse effect on plasma triglycerides[29].

With awareness of the association between unopposed estrogens and endometrial carcinoma, such treatment is no longer widely used unless a hysterectomy has been performed. As a result, there has been much concern that the beneficial changes in the lipid profile due to estrogen replacement may be partially reversed by the addition of progestogens[30]. All commercially available hormone replacement therapy calendar pack preparations contain testosterone-derived or C-19-derived progestogens for at least 10 and usually 12 days each month. C-19-derived progestogens were thought to convey a greater adverse effect on lipid profiles than C-21 derivatives; however, this study compared high doses of norethisterone acetate (10 mg) and norgestrel (0.5 mg) to the standard doses (10 mg) of medroxyprogesterone acetate[30]. It is now apparent that, if equivalent doses for endometrial transformation are given, the metabolic effects are similar[31]. More recently, epidemiological studies have indicated that relatively small doses of progestogens given for endometrial protection do not have significant negative effects on mortality[32].

The direct effect of estrogen on the female cardiovascular system is creating great interest. It has been shown that resistance to blood flow within the uterine and carotid arteries is reduced by estrogen within a few weeks of commencing treatment, and that, interestingly, the greater the interval between the menopause and the start of treatment the greater the effect[18]. It is postulated that this effect may be of equivalent or possibly even greater importance than the effect of hormone replacement therapy on lipids in the reduction of cardiovascular disease risk.

Potential risks of hormone replacement therapy

Despite the clearly documented benefits of hormone replacement therapy and the high proportion of women who suffer symptoms of the menopause, still only 8–10% of women in the United Kingdom are using hormone replacement therapy. Many women still perceive that to take hormone replacement therapy is to interfere with a natural process and that this in itself will lead to other as yet undiscovered risks. Many fear that use of exogenous estrogens will increase their risk of developing cancer. Others equate the risks to those of the combined oral contraceptive pill, advocating avoidance of hormone replacement therapy by women with a history of hypertension or thrombosis. However, the combined oral contraceptive pill contains the much more potent, synthetic estrogen ethinylestradiol and its effects cannot be compared to the natural estrogens used in estrogen replacement therapy.

Endometrial cancer

In the early 1970s, the increased risk of endometrial hyperplasia with unopposed estrogen therapy became apparent. The more atypical forms of endometrial hyperplasia may progress to endometrial carcinoma in up to 45% of cases. The use of unopposed estrogens with an intact uterus is associated with a 18–30% incidence of endometrial hyperplasia. The addition of at least 12 days' therapy with progestogens per cycle[33] has removed this problem, but public anxiety about hormone replacement therapy and its long-term risks remains. Additionally, a small proportion of patients will experience physical and psychological side-effects with progestogen addition which may deter its use. The side-effects include headaches, breast tenderness, bloating, anxiety and mood swings. However, these may be reduced by changing the progestogen type. Commercially available progestogens are C-19 nortestosterone derivatives (norethisterone, norgestrel), which tend to produce mildly androgenic side-effects such as greasy skin and hair and acne, and C-21 derivatives (medroxyprogesterone acetate, dydrogesterone), which in our experience are associated with depression and anxiety.

Pure progesterone can be given as suppositories or pessaries, but generally these routes of administration are not acceptable. Drowsiness is a side-effect associated with this therapy. When prescribing continuous bone-conserving doses of estrogen (see above), the usual doses of progestogens for secretory transformation of the endometrium are shown in Table 2.

Table 2   Daily doses of progestogens for secretory transformation of the endometrium

Norethisterone	0.7–1 mg
Norgestrel	0.15 mg
Dydrogesterone	10–20 mg
Medroxyprogesterone acetate	10 mg

A withdrawal bleed will usually occur at or shortly after the end of progestogen administration. A correlation between day of onset of bleeding and endometrial histology when using 12 days of progestogen administration each month has reduced the need for endometrial sampling. Padwick and co-workers[34] showed that, when bleeding occurred on or after the 11th day of progestogen administration, secretory endometrium was found in all patients studied. Bleeding before this time was associated with an inadequate progestogen effect and an increase in progestogen could correct the bleeding pattern. Hence the need for endometrial biopsy can now be confined to those women with persistent early or irregular bleeding.

At present, research is underway to develop continuous combined administration of estrogen and progestogen in regimens which will avoid withdrawal bleeds by inducing endometrial atrophy. Until their use is established, such regimens require endometrial biopsies on an annual basis as long-term safety data are not yet available. Detailed studies of the effects of these treatments on metabolic parameters are also awaited, although preliminary data look encouraging[35].

A new steroid, tibolone (Organon, Oss, Holland), which combines estrogenic, progestogenic and androgenic properties, has recently become available. This compound has many of the advantages of estrogen, without causing withdrawal bleeds in women more than 12 months postmenopausal. Comprehensive metabolic studies of this preparation are needed.

Breast cancer

The average woman in the UK has a 1 in 12 lifetime risk of developing breast carcinoma. Although there is still no agreement on the effect of hormone replacement therapy on breast cancer risk, nevertheless any further increase in risk would clearly be highly undesirable. Breast cancer appears to be a hormone-related malignancy; the risk increases with early menarche and late menopause, and decreases with late menarche and premature menopause. Many epidemiological studies have attempted to unravel the confusion which exists over the effect of estrogen replacement on breast cancer risk, to enable medical practitioners to provide more definite information to patients considering hormone replacement therapy.

Although many of the early studies were methodologically flawed because of small numbers and inclusion bias, there have been several well-designed studies over the last 12 years. Three[36–38] reported an increased risk in users with a history of surgically proven benign breast disease, whereas others[39,40] have not. In addition, the histological diagnosis of benign breast disease appears predictive, with those demonstrating atypia or epitheliosis being most at risk.

Others have attempted to correlate duration and dose of estrogen replacement with risk. Four studies[38,41–43] showed a moderate overall increase in relative risk (1.3–1.9) with 10 years or more of estrogen usage, and, of these, three reported an increase in risk with increasing dose[38,42,43]. However, three others[44–46] reported no increased risk with either dose or duration. More recently, the data from the Nurses' Health Study[47] showed a significant increase in risk for current users of hormone replacement therapy as compared to past users and this was due to increased duration of use (> 10 years).

Other factors which may influence risk are a family history (first-degree relative affected by the disease), type of menopause (natural or surgical) and history of hysterectomy. However, although there is no consensus at present on the use of hormone replacement therapy and breast cancer risk, clearly the risk of breast cancer is already high and, more importantly, the mortality rate in the UK is also high. General agreement exists that small doses of estrogen (conjugated equine estrogen 0.625 mg, estradiol valerate 2 mg, transdermal 17β-estradiol 50 μg) for short periods of time (up to 5 years) confer no significant increase in risk.

The effect of progestogens on breast tissue has recently been studied. Although they suppress mitoses in endometrium, they do not appear to have the same effect on breast tissue. Histological data[48] have suggested that progestogens may in fact increase the rate of cell turnover in breast tissue. A recent consensus conference stated that there was no evidence that the addition of progestogens to estrogen replacement in women who have undergone hysterectomy was justified.

Other diseases and hormone replacement therapy

Ovarian cancer

Although early studies suggested an increase in risk of endometrioid ovarian carcinoma with hormone replacement therapy, this evidence has since been attributed to bias due to study design. Results of recent reliable studies have not shown any increase in risk of any type of ovarian carcinoma. However, as ovarian carcinoma increases in frequency after the menopause, this is an ideal time to arrange screening in high-risk groups.

Cervical cancer

Hormone replacement therapy is not associated with an increased risk of carcinoma of the cervix, and there is no evidence that progression from premalignant to malignant disease is accelerated by therapy. Therefore previously abnormal smears or cervical carcinoma are not contraindications to use of hormone replacement therapy.

Hypertension

Blood pressure is not affected by hormone replacement therapy in the majority of women. In a minority taking oral estrogens (approximately 2%), blood pressure may rise, but this has been related to weight gain in these individuals. Otherwise, blood pressure does not increase; indeed, due to the direct effect upon blood vessels previously described, there may be a small fall in blood pressure. Despite warnings in Data Sheets, there is no evidence that well controlled hypertension should be considered a contraindication. Indeed, data are available that estrogens reduce risk of death from myocardial infarction in hypertensives.

Thromboembolism

Natural estrogens in the standard doses used in hormone replacement therapy do not appear to cause any clinically relevant changes in coagulation and fibrinolytic factors, and do not increase the risk of venous thromboembolism in apparently healthy women. If thrombosis were associated with an increase in estradiol levels, then there would be a higher incidence premenopausally, especially mid-cycle when estradiol levels are at their maximum and much higher than the levels achieved with standard doses of hormone replacement therapy. Nevertheless, there may be susceptible individuals, particularly those with antithrombin III deficiency or abnormal protein C levels, who are at an already higher risk of thrombosis. In these women, a sudden increase in plasma estradiol *may* increase the risk of thrombosis. Thus, in susceptible individuals with a relevant history, it may be advisable to monitor clotting factors before starting hormone replacement therapy. Additionally, a non-oral route of administration is less likely adversely to affect fibrinolytic coagulation profiles.

Gall bladder disease

Hormone replacement therapy increases the turnover of cholesterol in bile. An increase in risk of gall bladder disease has been identified with both oral contraceptive use and oral estrogen replacement therapy[49].

Endometriosis

Endometriosis is an estrogen-dependent disease which may be reactivated by hormone replacement therapy. Patients with endometriosis should be carefully monitored. In those patients who have undergone complete excision of the disease, the potential for recurrence is small but, nevertheless, may occasionally happen due to reactivation of micro-deposits.

Fibroids

Identical comments apply as for endometriosis, except that hysterectomy removes the risk of recurrence.

Contraindications to hormone replacement therapy

A recent history of breast cancer or well differentiated endometrial cancer beyond stage 1C (invasion greater than half of the myometrial thickness) are generally considered contraindications to hormone replacement therapy. However, there are currently very little data on the consequences of treating such patients with hormone replacement therapy, mainly because so few patients, having undergone surgery for this type of malignancy, would risk the possibility of it recurring.

Otosclerosis and systemic lupus erythematosis are conditions which may worsen in pregnancy, but they are rare and, therefore, there are little data on the effect of hormone replacement therapy. Additionally, isolated cases of systemic lupus erythematosis have been reported to improve in pregnancy. Therefore, it is advisable to be aware of signs of recurrence whilst hormone replacement therapy is being used,

Hypertension, thrombosis, diabetes and liver disease are not contraindications to hormone replacement therapy, although their management should carry special precautions such as closer monitoring. Risks of varicose veins are not affected by administration of hormone replacement therapy.

Abdominal vaginal bleeding must be investigated prior to use of hormone replacement therapy.

Pregnancy is always cited as a contraindication, but must be very uncommon in the typical menopausal age group!

Route of administration

All types of estrogen therapy will relieve symptoms of the menopause when adequate levels of estrogen are attained. However, the metabolic effects of estrogen may be influenced by the route of administration. During the fertile premenopausal years, the ovary principally produces estradiol. Estrone is produced from peripheral conversion of androstenedione in body fat, muscle and adrenals. In the postmenopausal years, therefore, there is very little natural production of estradiol, the female relying on the extra-ovarian production of estrone.

Estradiol given orally (estradiol valerate, micronized estradiol) is subjected to metabolism in the gut wall and liver; between 35%[50] and 60%[51] is converted to estrone glucuronide, which is inactive. This has several consequences. First, the dominant estrogen produced will be estrone. Additionally, in order to achieve adequate symptom relief, there must be a relative overdose of oral estrogens, depending upon the individual metabolism. Because there is a wide variation between individuals in the rate of absorption from the bowel, different patients may achieve different plasma levels despite identical doses. Finally, this first-pass hepatic effect may theoretically produce adverse changes in the production of certain hepatic proteins, such as renin substrate and clotting factors. In practice this has not been shown to influence clinical disease risk. Oral estrogens may also produce nausea and dyspepsia in some patients. The advantage of the oral route is that HDL-cholesterol is elevated more than with equivalent non-oral estrogen delivery systems.

Non-oral estrogens may be given vaginally (estriol), transdermally (17β-estradiol patch) or subcutaneously (estradiol implant).

Transdermal and implant therapy avoid the first-pass hepatic effect and primarily deliver estradiol into the plasma, therefore more closely mimicking the premenopausal environment. The smaller degree of degradation means that smaller doses of estrogen can be administered in order to achieve similar symptom relief to that seen with the higher doses of oral estrogen. However, transdermal and implant therapies also have their disadvantages. Patches may cause irritation, occurring in around 20–30% of women, and this may be so severe as to cause blisters, even in women with no previous history of skin reactions. Implants require a surgical procedure every 6 months. This may lead to a steady increase in estradiol levels, seen with subsequent implants and associated with earlier and earlier recurrence of symptoms and earlier requests for repeat implants by the patient (tachyphylaxis). Although this occurs in a small proportion of patients using implant therapy, nevertheless, it is a distressing condition and it is important to avoid it by strict adherence to timing of implants at no more than 6-monthly intervals and/or monitoring of estradiol levels. Overall, however, one route of administration will be acceptable to the majority of patients, although certain conditions may point to one route being more acceptable or desirable for 'at-risk' patients, e.g. the non-oral route when risk of venous thrombosis is increased.

Conclusion

More women are becoming aware about the some-
times devastating consequences of the untreated
menopause. Clearly, quite apart from the relief of
menopausal symptoms, the long-term benefits of
hormone replacement therapy are considerable, both
in the reduction of osteoporosis and cardiovascular
disease risk. Each individual should have access to a
doctor to discuss her relative risks from these conditions in order to make an informed decision as to
whether this treatment would be appropriate for her.

Section 2   The Menopause Illustrated

List of illustrations

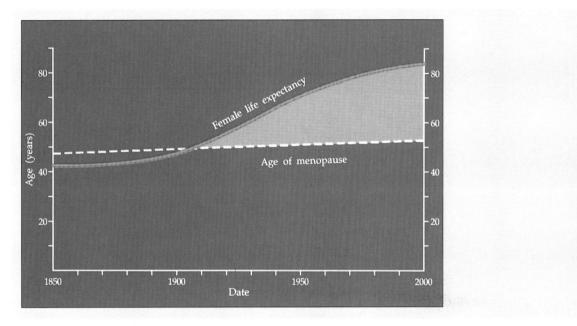

Figure 1 Female life expectancy plotted against age at menopause from 1850 projected through to the year 2000. Whereas the age of menopause has changed but little, the female life expectancy has increased and is currently approximately 80 years. The average woman can expect to spend one-third of her life in a postmenopausal state[52]

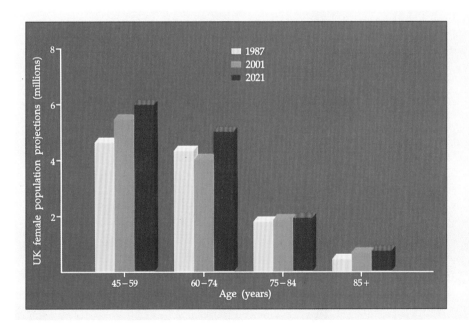

Figure 2 Female population in the United Kingdom in defined age bands in 1987 and projected to the years 2001 and 2021. Note increased numbers in all age bands projected over the next 35 years which will place an increasing strain on health care resources[53]

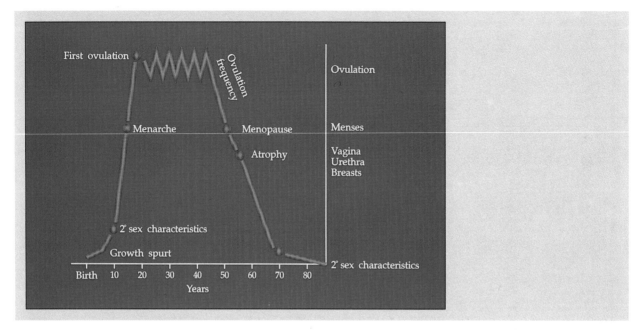

Figure 3 Schematic representation of estradiol values during the female lifespan assuming menarche around age 14 years and menopause around age 51 years. Estradiol production increases markedly during puberty and fluctuates cyclically during the reproductive era. Estradiol production may decline in the years immediately preceding menopause and typical estrogen-deficiency symptoms (such as flushes and sweats) may first arise during this time. When the plasma values are no longer above the threshold for endometrial stimulation, menstruation ceases. Intermittent ovarian activity can occur postmenopausally and thus the plasma values may not fall abruptly immediately following the last period. Thus, the menopause is but one marker in the continuum of declining ovarian activity[54]

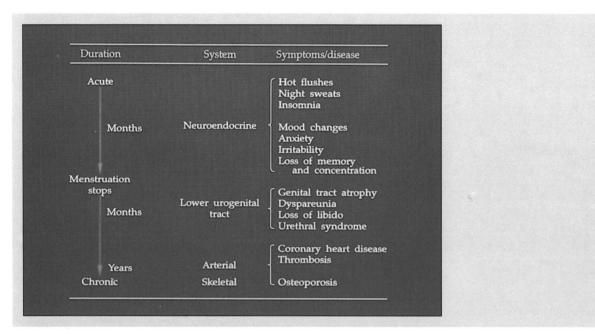

Figure 4 Acute and chronic sequelae of ovarian failure and their temporal relationship with cessation of menstruation. Because estradiol receptors have been identified in many tissues throughout the body, the sequelae of estrogen deficiency involve a wide spectrum of target organs. Neuroendocrine symptoms often arise in the perimenopause. Those due to lower genital tract atrophy may also arise at this time but, in our experience, usually only become sufficiently severe to warrant medical intervention after menopause. The major causes of morbidity and mortality, osteoporosis and coronary heart disease, may not arise until many years after menopause[55]

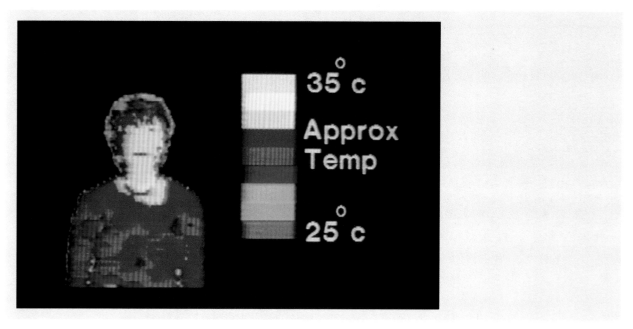

Figure 5 Skin temperature, as measured by thermography, over the head, neck and thorax of a postmenopausal woman immediately prior to a hot flush. The skin temperature at these sites varies as indicated by the different colors

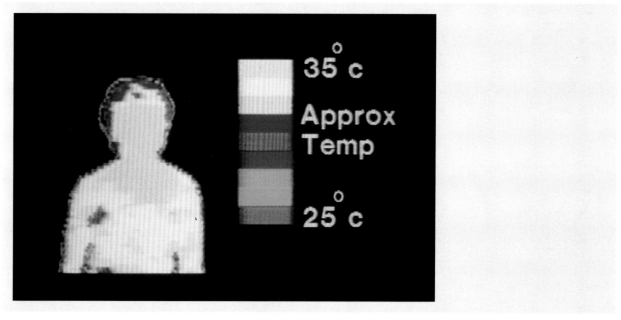

Figure 6 Thermogram of the same woman taken some minutes later at the height of a hot flush. The marked color changes indicate a rise in skin temperature due to vasodilatation. Patients usually complain that flushes particularly affect the face and neck but the thermogram demonstrates that similar changes occur over the thoracic region as well

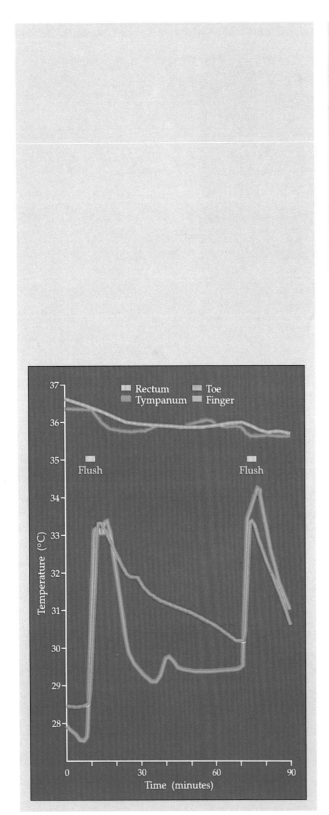

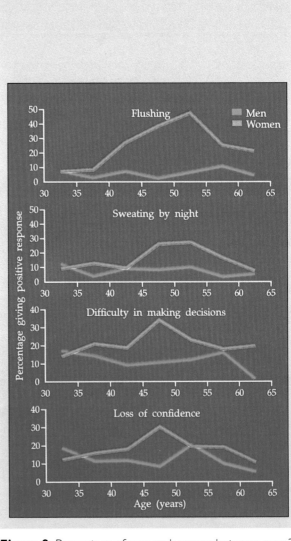

Figure 7 Changes in peripheral (finger and toe) and central (core) temperatures (rectum and tympanum) in a postmenopausal woman who experienced two flushes over a 90-min period of observation. The marked rises in peripheral temperature were followed by small falls in core temperature. The changes in finger and toe temperature with the flushing episodes demonstrate that flushes cause generalized vascular phenomena[56]

Figure 8 Percentage of men and women between ages 30 and 65 years reporting various symptoms by postal questionnaire. No mention of the true nature of this survey – to identify symptoms associated with the climacteric – was included in the questionnaire. The percentage of women with flushes increased markedly from age 40 years and a similar rise was observed with sweating by night. The percentage of women reporting difficulty in making decisions and loss of confidence doubled around the climacteric[3]

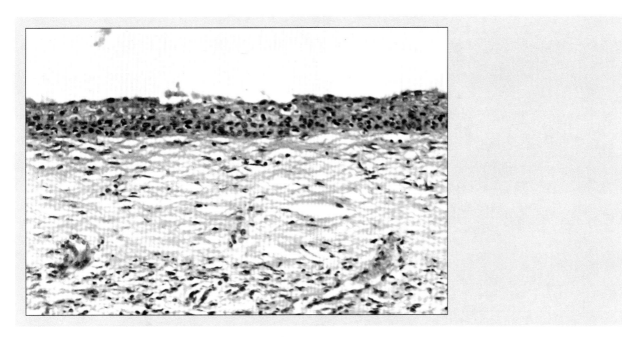

Figure 9 Cross-section of the vaginal epithelium from a premenopausal woman. The classic description is of an epithelium divided into basal, intermediate and superficial layers. Each is many cells thick

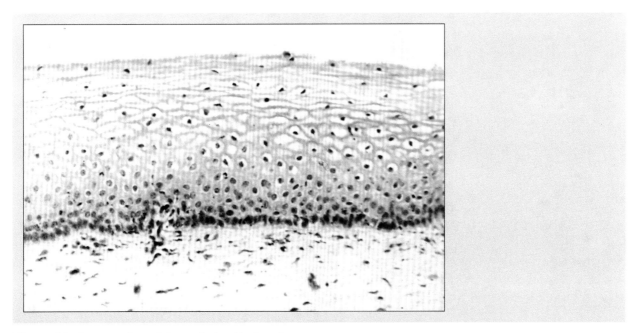

Figure 10 Cross-section of the vaginal epithelium from a postmenopausal woman. Following loss of estradiol, the epithelium thins and all cell layers are involved. There is a progressive decrease in vascularity of the underlying tissues and a gradual loss of elastin and collagen. The vaginal skin becomes pale and fragile with increased predisposition to bacterial infection

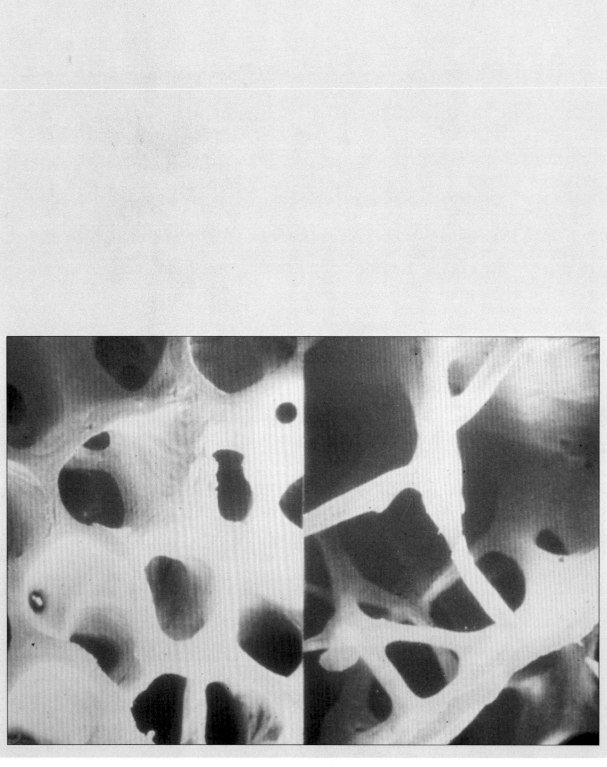

Figure 11 Scanning electron photomicrograph of normal (left) trabecular bone from a premenopausal woman and osteoporotic (right) trabecular bone from a postmenopausal woman. The normal bone contains a matrix of thick trabeculae in a honeycomb distribution. Loss of bony tissue leads to thinning of the trabeculae which reduces bone strength and increases the risk of fracture[57]

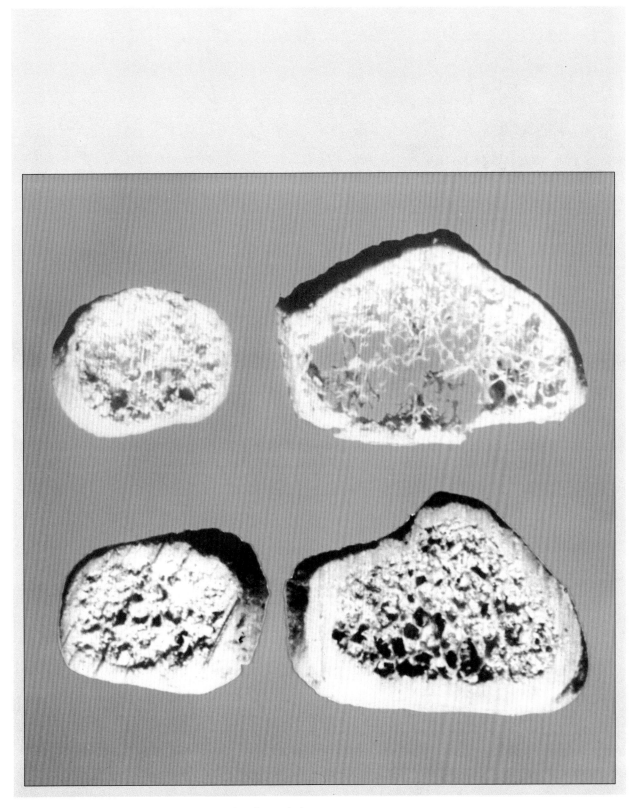

Figure 12 Cross-section through the distal radius and ulna of a 70-year-old woman (top) and a 70-year-old man (bottom). The distal radius and ulna have a relatively high proportion of trabecular as compared to cortical bone. Note loss of both types of bone in the woman as compared to the man. This loss increases the risk of fracture (Figure 14) and explains why this fracture occurs so much more commonly in women as compared to men (Figure 15)

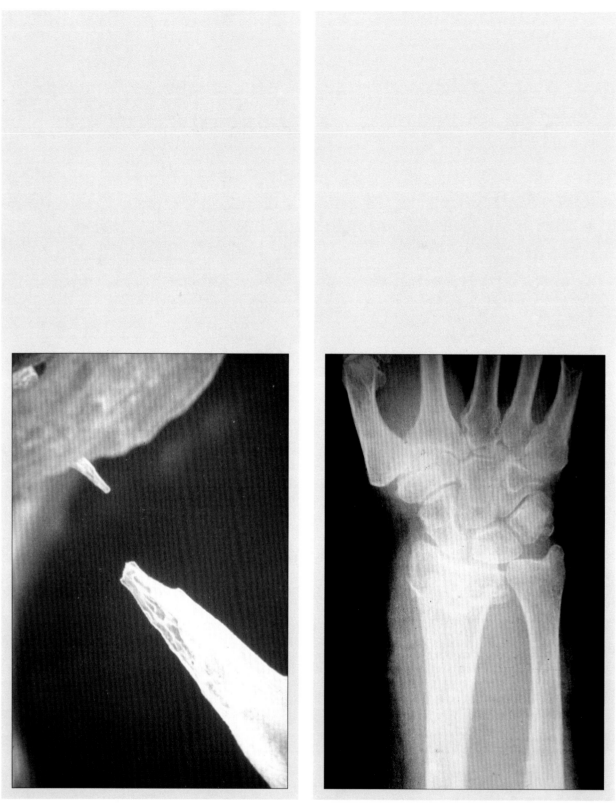

Figure 13 Scanning electron photomicrograph from an osteoporotic woman showing microfracture of a bony trabeculum. Resorption pits from excessive osteoclastic activity can be clearly seen. This microfracture illustrates why advanced osteoporotic damage may not respond well to treatments such as hormone replacement therapy, the calcitonins and the bisphosphonates. All of these treatments work primarily by decreasing bone resorption: they do not encourage reanastomosis of trabecular fragments[57]

Figure 14 Radiograph showing distal radius (Colles') fracture. The distal radius is one of the three sites for classical osteoporotic fracture. It contains a relatively high proportion of trabecular bone. Fracture usually occurs, often in the nondominant wrist, when the arm is outstretched as a protective mechanism against a forward fall

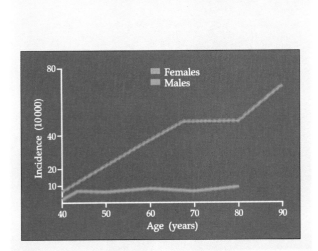

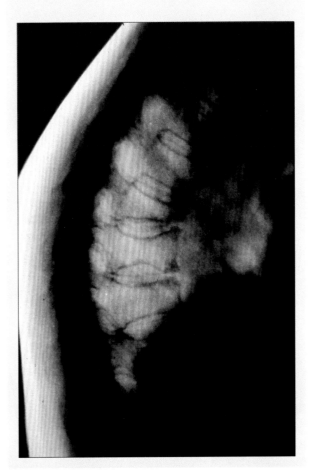

Figure 15 Incidence of Colles' fracture in females as compared to males per 10 000 population between ages 40 and 80 years. The rate of increase is much higher in females than in males

Figure 16 Radiograph showing wedging of thoracic vertebrae. The anterior aspect of the vertebral body is affected more than the posterior part by osteoporosis, and the former is gradually compressed leading to kyphosis. Estimates for the incidence of vertebral wedging vary widely, largely because different authors have used dissimilar criteria for diagnosing the condition. However, it is generally accepted that at least 12–15% of women suffer vertebral wedging during their sixties and this figure rises to around 25% in the eighth decade

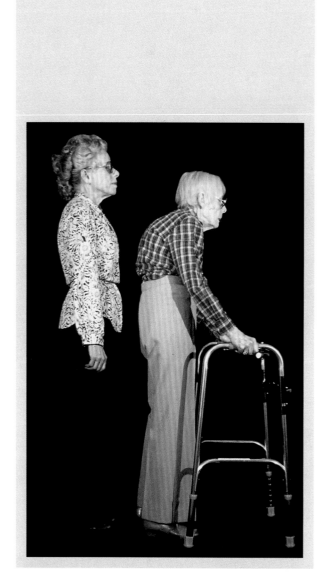

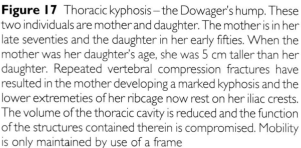

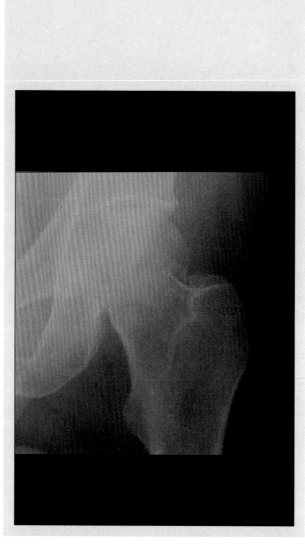

Figure 17 Thoracic kyphosis – the Dowager's hump. These two individuals are mother and daughter. The mother is in her late seventies and the daughter in her early fifties. When the mother was her daughter's age, she was 5 cm taller than her daughter. Repeated vertebral compression fractures have resulted in the mother developing a marked kyphosis and the lower extremeties of her ribcage now rest on her iliac crests. The volume of the thoracic cavity is reduced and the function of the structures contained therein is compromised. Mobility is only maintained by use of a frame

Figure 18 Radiograph showing fracture of the proximal femur. In the United Kingdom, this fracture ranks third in the list of use of hospital beds for non-psychiatric purposes. The associated mortality is high with approximately 15–20% of women succumbing in direct consequence. Morbidity is also considerable: less than one-half of women with this fracture are able to return to a 'normal' life. Many require sheltered accommodation. The incidence of fracture of the proximal femur rises sharply after age 70 years, doubling every 5 years. By the ninth decade, one woman in three will suffer this fracture

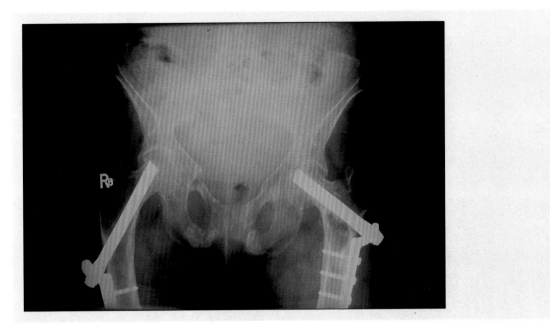

Figure 19 Severe postmenopausal osteoporosis has led to fracture of both hips, requiring surgery. The prognosis for elderly women with hip fracture has to be guarded. Between 15 and 20% of women with this fracture die as a direct consequence, and 25–50% of those who survive never regain full mobility

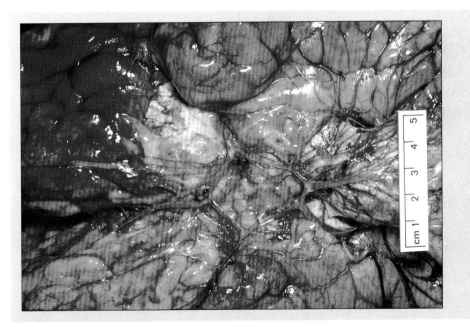

Figure 20 Cerebral infarct: progressive atherosclerosis of the cerebral vessels increases the risk of cerebrovascular accident. The incidence is influenced by some of the same risk factors as for myocardial infarction

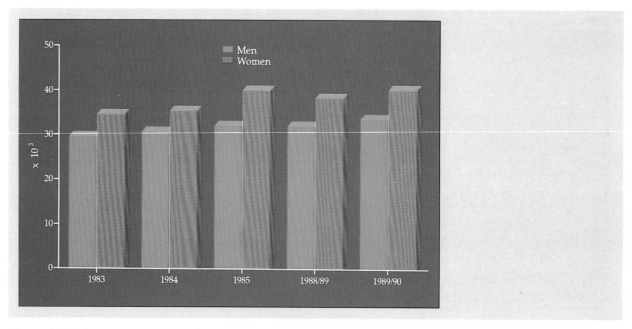

Figure 21 Estimated numbers ($\times 10^3$) of men and women with ICD436 (cerebrovascular accident) between 1983 and 1990. This diagnosis is made more commonly in women than in men[58]

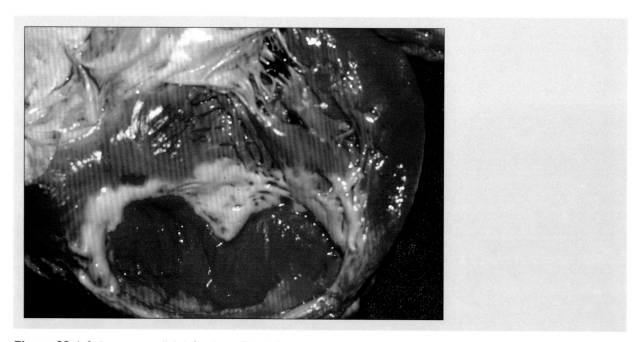

Figure 22 Inferior myocardial infarction. The infarcted tissue is necrotic and the myocardial tissue around it has become white due to ischemia. Overall, cardiovascular disease remains the leading cause of death in women. It is relatively uncommon premenopausally but increases dramatically in incidence postmenopausally (see Figure 35)

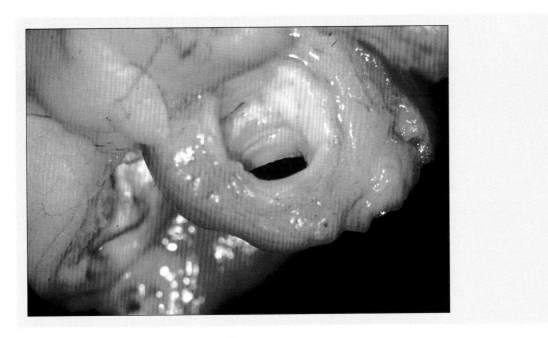

Figure 23 Atheromatous coronary arteries

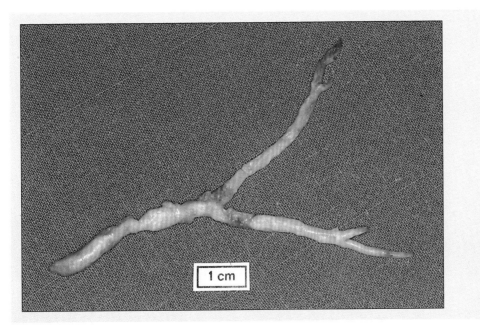

Figure 24 Dissected atheromatous coronary arteries. The vessel walls are diseased with loss of elasticity. The lumen is reduced and partially obstructed at numerous sites by atheromatous plaque

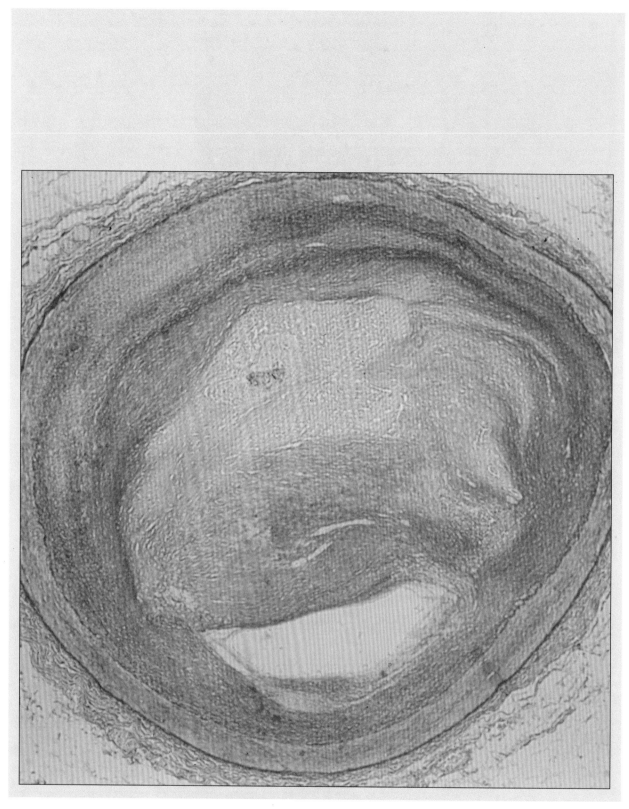

Figure 25 Cross-section through a medium-sized coronary artery showing almost complete occlusion by atheromatous plaque

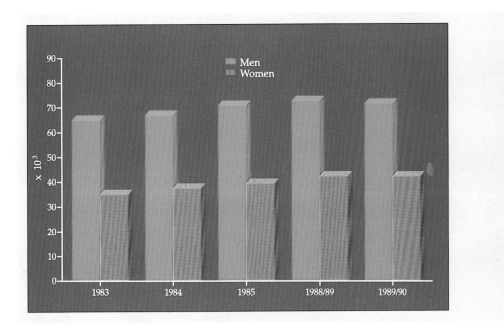

Figure 26 Estimated numbers ($\times 10^3$) of men and women with ICD410 (myocardial infarction) between 1983 and 1990[58]

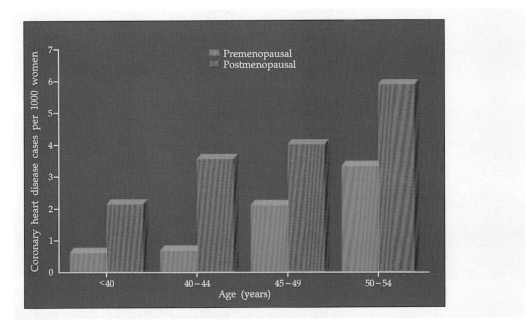

Figure 27 Incidence of coronary heart disease per 1000 women in defined age bands and according to menopausal status. In both pre- and postmenopausal women the incidence increases with advancing age. However, within each age band loss of ovarian function is associated with a higher risk of coronary heart disease[11]

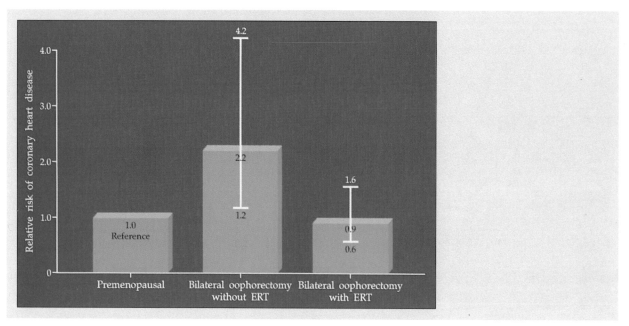

Figure 28 Relative risk of coronary heart disease in the Nurses' Health Study. In premenopausal women the relative risk was standardized to 1.0. Early bilateral oophorectomy without subsequent use of ERT (estrogen replacement therapy) was associated with a relative risk of 2.2. Early bilateral oophorectomy followed by use of ERT was associated with a relative risk of 0.9. 95% confidence intervals are as shown. Data are adjusted for age and smoking[59]

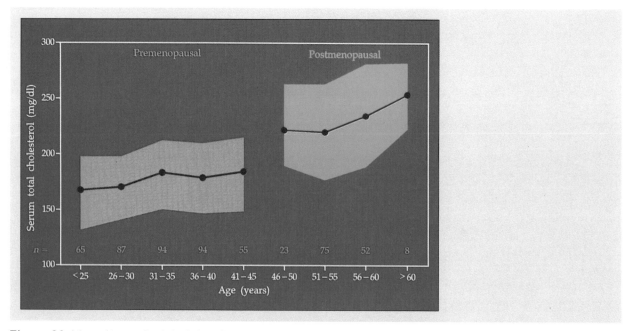

Figure 29 Mean (± standard deviation, SD) total cholesterol levels in women by 5-year age bands from less than 25 years old to greater than 60 years old. Data are adjusted for body mass index, gravidity, smoking and exercise and observations from women with thyroid disease have been excluded. Note the profound effects of loss of endogenous estradiol on total cholesterol levels. n = number of observations in each age band[60]

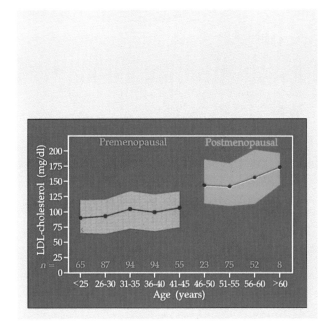

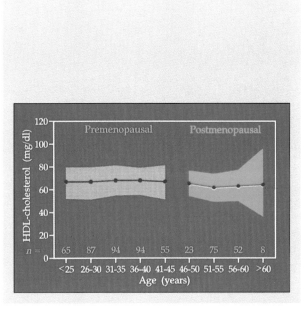

Figure 30 Mean (± SD) low density lipoprotein (LDL)-cholesterol levels in same women as in Figure 29. The rise in total cholesterol at menopause shown in Figure 29 is explained, in this Figure, by an increase in the potentially atherogenic LDL subfraction[60]

Figure 31 Mean (± SD) high density lipoprotein (HDL)-cholesterol levels in same women. Loss of endogenous estradiol at menopause has little effect upon HDL-cholesterol[60]

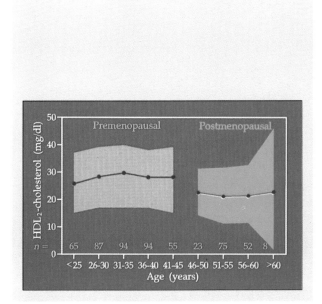

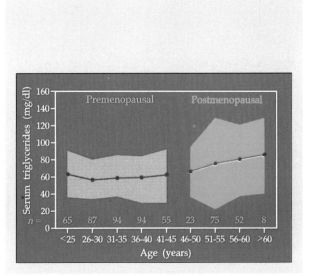

Figure 32 Mean (± SD) HDL$_2$-cholesterol levels in same women. Loss of endogenous estradiol at menopause is associated with reduction in HDL$_2$-cholesterol, which is thought to be cardioprotective. Lower HDL$_2$-cholesterol values with higher LDL-cholesterol levels (Figure 30) may explain the increased risk of coronary heart disease seen after menopause. Comparison with Figure 31 illustrates the limited value of 'total' HDL-cholesterol measurements. These may not change, yet important alterations may be occurring in clinically relevant HDL subfractions[60]

Figure 33 Mean (± standard deviation) triglyceride levels in same women. Because triglyceride data are not normally distributed, the results were log-transformed prior to analysis. The rise in triglycerides in the postmenopausal women appeared more age-related than due to loss of endogenous estradiol[60]

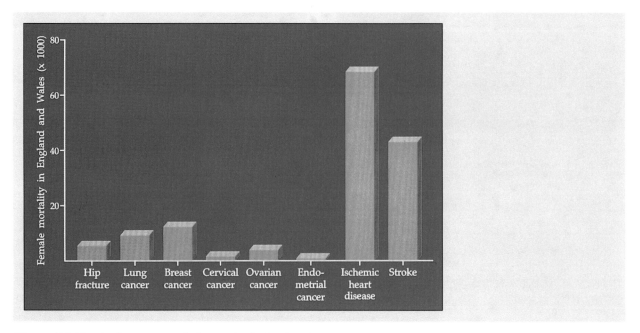

Figure 34 Deaths in women of all ages in England and Wales by selected underlying causes in 1987. Deaths from hip fractures are estimated. Deaths from ischemic heart disease and stroke greatly outnumber deaths from all gynecological malignancies, lung cancer and hip fracture combined[61,62]

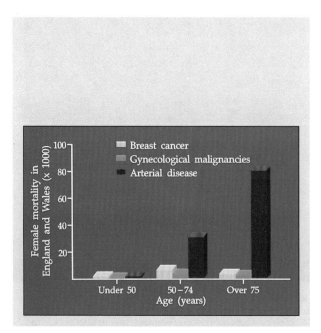

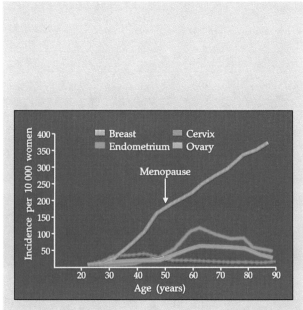

Figure 35 Deaths in women from breast cancer, gynecological malignancies and arterial disease according to age group, in England and Wales in 1987. Note: 'gynecological malignancies' include adnexal neoplasms; arterial disease includes deaths from ischemic heart disease and cerebrovascular disease. Under 50 years of age, the numbers of deaths from these three conditions are similar. However, deaths from arterial disease rise much more rapidly after age 50 years[61]

Figure 36 Incidence of various gynecological malignancies per 100 000 women aged 20–90 years. The rate of increase of breast carcinoma is greater than that of carcinoma of the cervix, endometrium or ovary between 30 and 45 years of age. Around the menopause, the rate of increase of breast carcinoma declines and it is suggested that the menopause may confer a degree of protection against breast carcinoma[63]

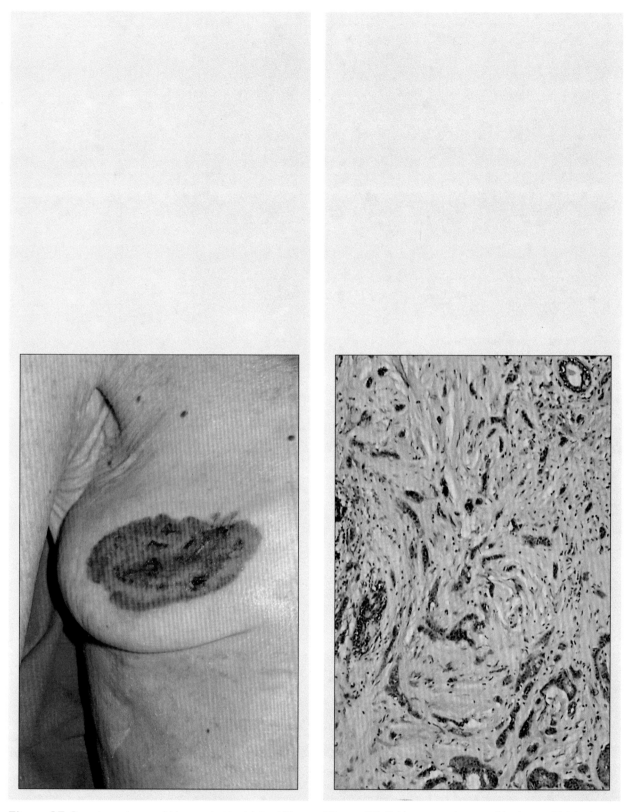

Figure 37 Breast carcinoma. Women in the United Kingdom have a 1 in 11 lifetime risk of developing breast cancer and mortality remains high. There is an increase in risk in women who undergo early menarche and/or late menopause. This suggests that duration of exposure to estrogen influences lifetime risk

Figure 38 Schirrous carcinoma of the breast. This is characterized by clumps of anaplastic, spheroidal carcinoma cells surrounded by bands of fibroid tissue. This is the commonest type of breast carcinoma

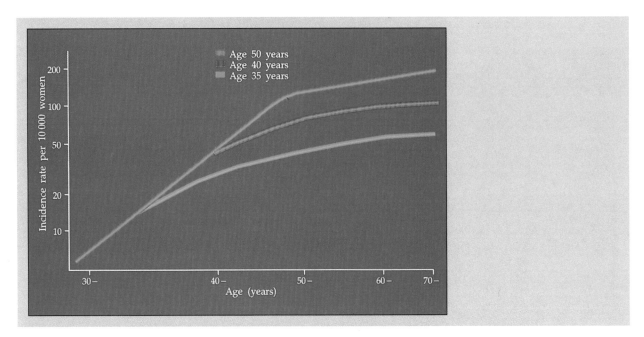

Figure 39 Age incidence curves for breast cancer per 100 000 women assuming menopause at age 50, 40 and 35 years. The protective effect of early menopause raises concerns that administration of exogenous estrogens will increase the risk of breast cancer[64]

Estrogen preparation	Follicle stimulating hormone	Cortisol binding globulin binding capacity	Sex hormone binding globulin binding capacity	Renin substrate
Piperazine estrone sulphate	1.0	1.0	1.0	1.0
Micronized estradiol	1.3	1.9	1.0	0.7
Conjugated equine estrogens	1.4	2.5	3.2	3.5
Diethylstilbestrol	3.8	70	28	13
Ethinylestradiol	80–200*	1000	614	232

Figure 40 Relative potencies of various natural and synthetic estrogens on suppression of follicle stimulating hormone and stimulation of certain hepatically derived proteins and globulins – cortisol binding globulin binding capacity, sex hormone binding globulin binding capacity, and renin substrate in postmenopausal women. The natural estrogens are piperazine estrone sulphate and micronized estradiol; synthetic estrogens are diethylstilbestrol and ethinylestradiol. Conjugated equine estrogens are a complex mixture of which approximately 60% is estrone sulphate. Results are expressed in milligram equivalents of piperazine estrone sulphate which has been ascribed a relative potency of 1.0. The synthetic estrogens have a much greater relative potency as compared to their natural counterparts. Thus, it is unwise to extrapolate risks observed with synthetic estrogens, as prescribed in the combined oral contraceptive pill, to use of natural estrogens in postmenopausal women. *Estimated in the absence of parallelism[65]

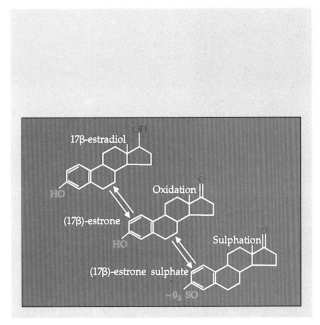

Figure 41 Schematic representation of intracellular metabolism of 17β-estradiol. The initial step is oxidation to estrone by the 17β-dehydrogenases. The next step is sulphation to estrone sulphate which is achieved by sulphatases. Estrone sulphate is water soluble and passes out of the cell into the interstitial fluid. Both of these enzymatic degradation steps are reversible but favor estradiol → estrone → estrone sulphate. Manipulation of the estradiol molecule and insertion of an ethinyl group at the C-17 position (to produce ethinylestradiol) means that this degradation cannot occur. The 17β-dehydrogenases cannot oxidize the hydroxyl group because of the covalent bond on carbon-17. As a result, the potency of ethinylestradiol is greatly enhanced (see Figure 40)

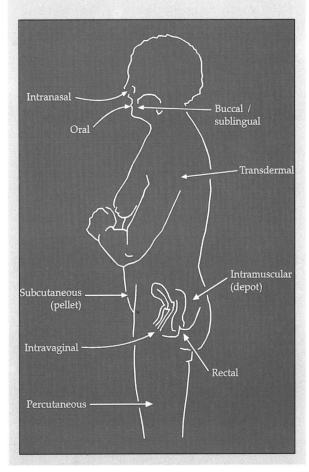

Figure 42 Potential routes of estrogen administration. In the United Kingdom, four routes are commonly used: oral, transdermal, subcutaneous (implant) and vaginal (tablet, pessary or cream). Other routes, such as sublingual and intranasal, have been investigated but the plasma half-life of estrogens delivered by these routes appears short and they are still being evaluated

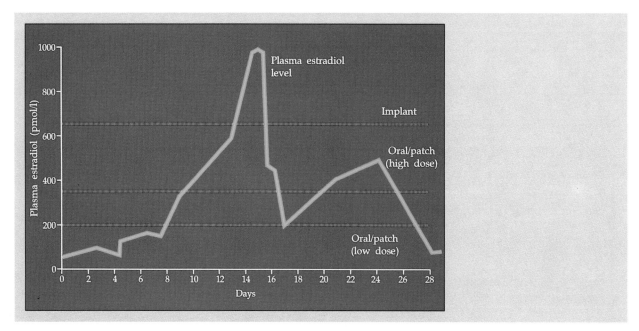

Figure 43 Schematic representation of the plasma estradiol values achieved with oral, transdermal and subcutaneous (implant) estrogen therapies. For comparative purposes, the estradiol levels observed during the menstrual cycle in the reproductive era have been included. Oral/patch (low-dose) is conjugated equine estrogens 0.625 mg/day or transdermal estradiol 50 µg/day. Oral/patch (high-dose) is conjugated equine estrogens 1.25 mg/day or transdermal estradiol 100 µg/day. The plasma estradiol value with implants was observed 6 months after the last implantation in a group of women receiving estradiol 50 mg at 6-monthly intervals. Oral/patch at low and high dose give plasma estradiol values less than the average value achieved during the normal ovulatory cycle (approximately 500 pmol/l)[66,67]

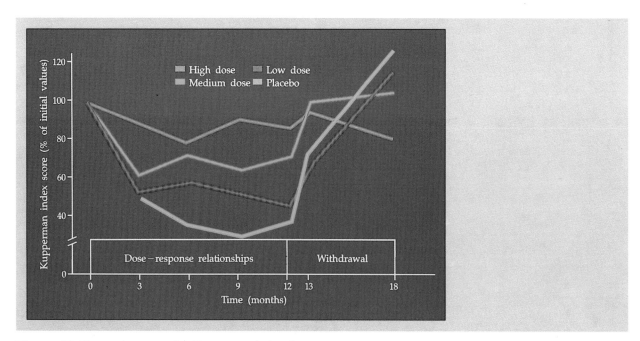

Figure 44 Change in scores for Kupperman index (sum score of 11 menopausal symptoms) in a blinded, placebo-controlled, dose-ranging study. High dose = estradiol 4 mg/day; medium dose = estradiol 2 mg/day; and low dose = estradiol 1 mg/day. Each dose was administered for 12 months and assessments were continued for 6 months after withdrawal of therapy. Kupperman index scores improved with therapy in a dose-dependent fashion[68]

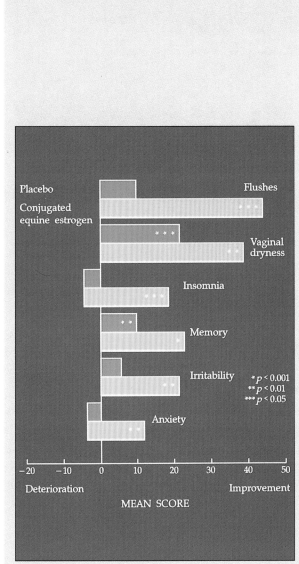

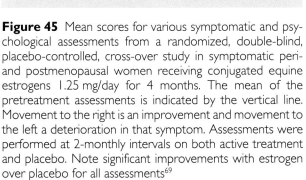

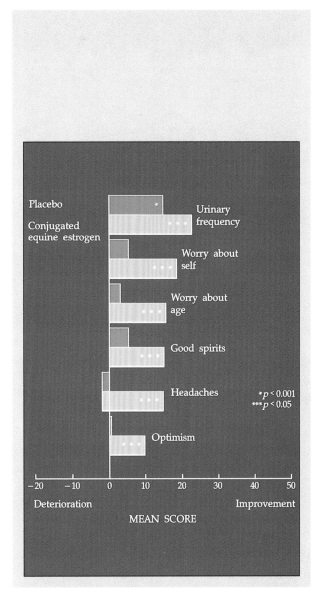

Figure 45 Mean scores for various symptomatic and psychological assessments from a randomized, double-blind, placebo-controlled, cross-over study in symptomatic peri- and postmenopausal women receiving conjugated equine estrogens 1.25 mg/day for 4 months. The mean of the pretreatment assessments is indicated by the vertical line. Movement to the right is an improvement and movement to the left a deterioration in that symptom. Assessments were performed at 2-monthly intervals on both active treatment and placebo. Note significant improvements with estrogen over placebo for all assessments[69]

Figure 46 Mean scores for various symptomatic and psychological assessments from the same study as in Figure 45. Note significant improvements with estrogen over placebo for all assessments. The authors suggested that the improvement in the psychological symptoms was due, in part, to a 'domino effect', with relief of daytime flushing and nocturnal sweating (and improvement in sleep pattern) causing a general feeling of well-being[69]

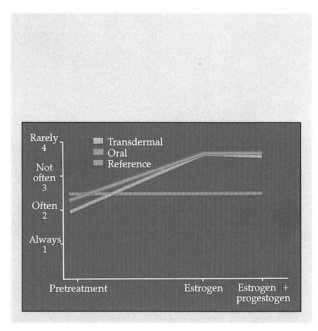

Figure 48 Median scores for hot flushes in three groups of early postmenopausal women, with 30 patients in each group, over a 3-month period. One group received transdermal estradiol 50 µg/day for 28 days with transdermal norethisterone acetate 0.25 mg/day added for 14 days each cycle. The second treated group received conjugated equine estrogens 0.625 mg/day in 28-day cycles with dl norgestrel 0.15 mg/day added for 12 days each cycle. Patients in the third group were not seeking hormone replacement therapy and were included as a reference group. Note similar beneficial effect upon the flushes in the two treated groups. On treatment assessments in third treatment cycle during estrogen-only and combined estrogen/progestogen phase

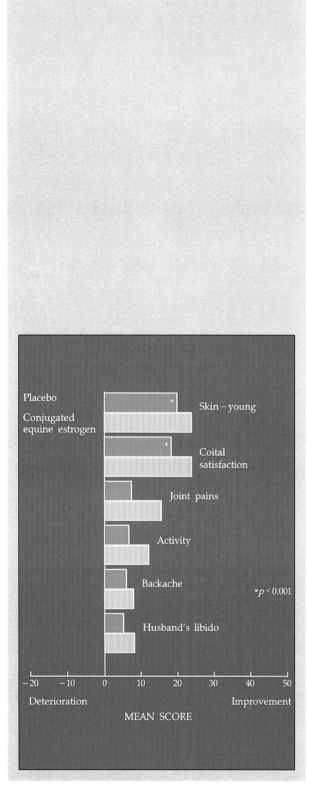

Figure 47 Mean scores for various symptomatic and psychological assessments from the same study as in Figure 45. Note marked placebo effect on youthful skin appearance and coital satisfaction[69]

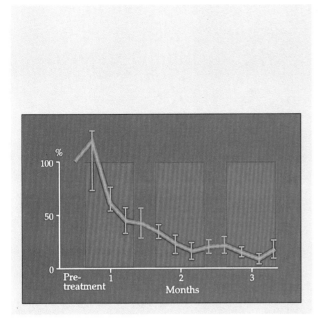

Figure 49 Percentage change in mean (± standard error) daily number of hot flushes during the first 3 months of therapy with cyclic transdermal estradiol 50 μg/day. The daily number of hot flushes had decreased by approximately 55% after the first 3-week course of treatment; by approximately 80% after the second treatment course, and by 91% at the end of the third course of treatment[70]

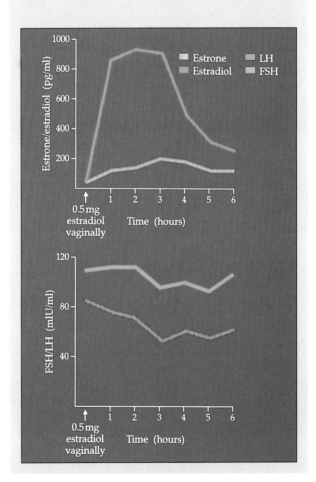

Figure 50 Plasma estrone, estradiol, luteinizing hormone (LH) and follicle stimulating hormone (FSH) levels after the vaginal administration of 0.5 mg micronized estradiol. Administration of estradiol results in a steep rise in the plasma estradiol level to a maximum of 800–900 pg/ml. This is maintained for 3 h after which there is a rapid decline. The estrone level rises more slowly to a maximum of approximately 200 pg/ml. The rise in estradiol corresponds with a suppression of LH of 37% at 180 min after estrogen administration and with a lesser suppression of FSH of around 13%. This was maximal at 3–5 h post-administration. Vaginal administration avoids the conversion of estradiol to estrone which occurs with oral estrogens within the gut wall. Hence, estradiol is transmitted directly into the systemic circulation. Therefore, vaginal administration of estradiol will produce a more physiological plasma estrogen profile than oral administration[71]

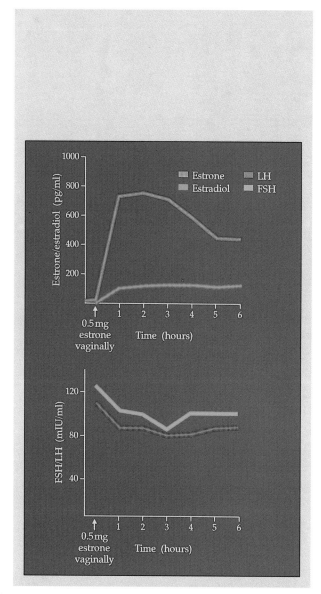

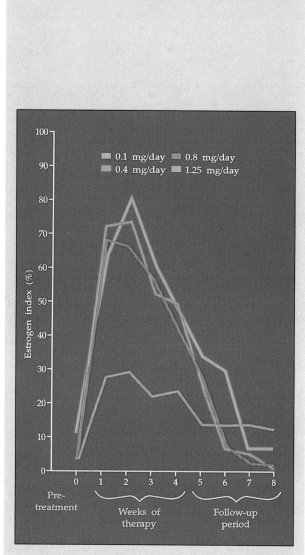

Figure 51 Plasma estrone, estradiol, luteinizing hormone (LH) and follicle stimulating hormone (FSH) levels after the vaginal administration of 0.5 mg estrone. There is a more pronounced rise in estrone to approximately 725 pg/ml by the first hour post-administration. This is maintained for 2 h whilst the rise in the estradiol level is less, to a maximum of approximately 100–135 pg/ml. There was a significant suppression of FSH and LH of 30% by 3 h and this was maintained for another 3 h. This and the previous figure illustrate that significant systemic absorption of estrogens occurs through the vaginal epithelium. Unless the estrogen dose is very small, it is therefore advisable that progestogens be added to the estrogen in women with an intact uterus. This and the previous figure also illustrate that, with vaginal administration, estradiol is absorbed as estradiol (Figure 50) and estrone as estrone (Figure 51)[71]

Figure 52 Effect of four different doses of vaginally administered conjugated equine estrogens (CEE) cream on the estrogen index of the vaginal epithelium. A total of 24 postmenopausal women received 2 g estrogen cream vaginally each night containing either 0.1 mg, 0.4 mg, 0.8 mg or 1.25 mg CEE. The estrogen index was measured cytologically pretreatment, weekly throughout the 4-week treatment phase, and weekly for a further 4 weeks after treatment had finished. All four doses produced premenopausal values for vaginal cytology. After treatment had been withdrawn, the estrogen index remained persistently above baseline only with the lowest dose. With the three higher doses the estrogen index reverted back to the postmenopausal range within 7 days. This may be explained by down-regulation of the estrogen receptors with the three higher doses[72]

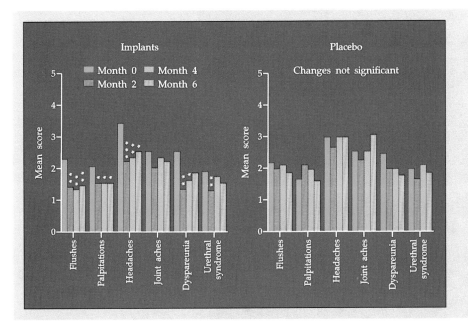

Figure 53 Effects of subcutaneous estradiol and testosterone implants on physical symptoms of the menopause. A total of 55 postmenopausal women requesting hormone replacement therapy for symptom relief were randomized in a double-blind manner to receive either estradiol 50 mg and testosterone 100 mg implants or placebo. Pretreatment they completed a questionnaire on the presence of physical symptoms. The questions were answered on a five-point scale where 5 indicated maximum symptom severity. The questionnaire was repeated 2, 4 and 6 months after treatment had been started. There was a significant improvement in all physical symptoms after 2 months of treatment with hormone implants as compared to placebo except for joint aches where the improvement was not significant[73]

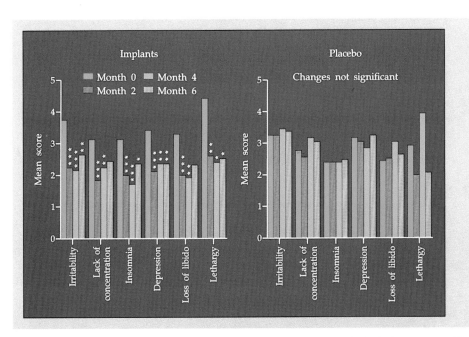

Figure 54 Effect of subcutaneous estradiol and testosterone implants on the psychological symptoms of the menopause. A total of 55 postmenopausal women requesting hormone replacement therapy for symptom relief were randomized in a double-blind manner to receive either estradiol 50 mg and testosterone 100 mg implants or placebo. Pretreatment they completed a questionnaire on psychological symptoms. The questions were answered on a five-point scale where 5 indicated maximum symptom severity. The questionnaire was repeated 2, 4 and 6 months after treatment had been started. All symptoms showed a marked improvement which was highly significant even after 2 months of active treatment. There was no improvement in the group receiving placebo[74]

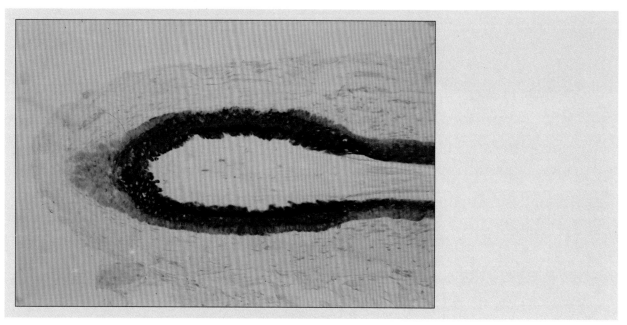

Figure 55 Transverse section through hair follicle stained with peroxidase for the presence of a protein associated with the estradiol receptor. This is indicated by the dense staining. Postmenopausal women frequently experience dry or thinning hair which is improved by HRT. The presence of an estradiol receptor within the hair follicle would explain this response to estrogen lack and replacement[75]

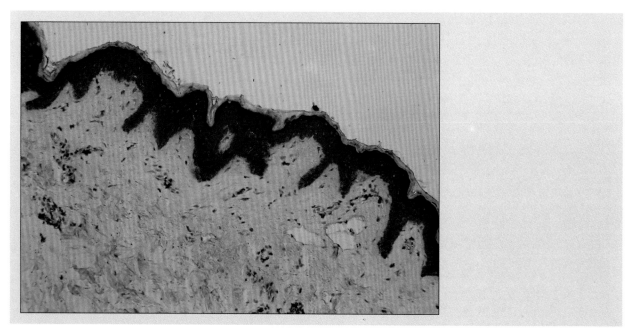

Figure 56 Staining for the presence of a protein associated with the estradiol receptor within the skin. The most intense staining is within the epidermis. The presence of this protein suggests that estrogen affects the skin. Dry, flaking, itching skin is commonly experienced postmenopausally, and an improvement may often be seen with estrogen replacement therapy[75]

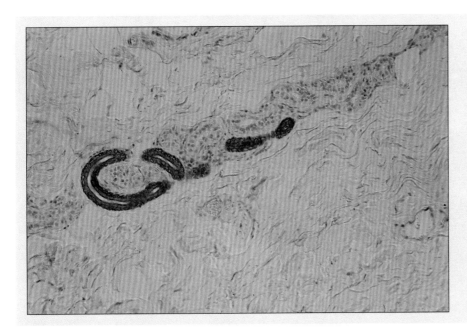

Figure 57 Staining for the presence of a protein associated with the estradiol receptor within a sebaceous gland. Staining was less dense than in the epidermis, but was present. This offers a further explanation for the dry texture of skin experienced by postmenopausal women[75]

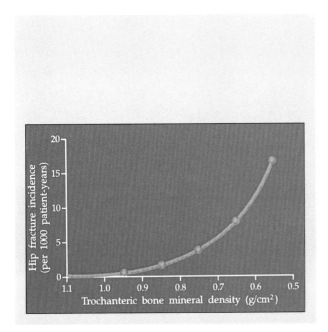

Figure 58 Relationship between the incidence of hip fracture and bone mineral density, as measured by dual photon absorptiometry in the femoral neck, in a population of women from Rochester, Minnesota, USA. The hip fracture rate increased as femoral bone density declined; few women experienced fracture when bone density was greater than 1.0 g/cm². However, the rate of increase in fracture incidence rose markedly when bone density fell below this figure. This emphasizes the importance of preventing further bone loss, even in those women who already have reduced bone density and are many years postmenopausal. Such women with reduced bone density should be offered treatments to stabilize the skeleton, prevent further bone loss and a further increase in fracture risk[76]

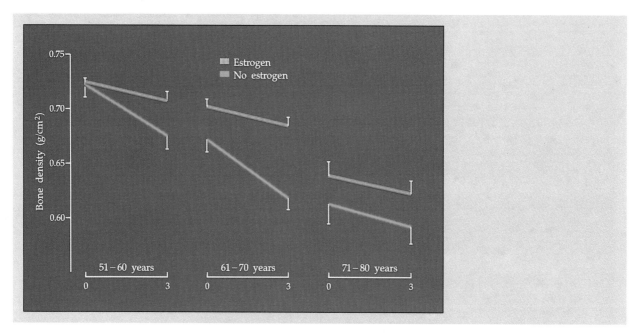

Figure 59 A comparison of the effects of estrogen replacement (micronized estradiol 1 mg daily, conjugated equine estrogens 0.625 mg daily) versus placebo on bone density, as determined with sequential measurements using single photon absorptiometry. Measurements of the distal radius were made over 3-year intervals in 397 postmenopausal women. They were divided into three age groups: 51–60 years, 61–70 years, 71–80 years. As compared to the untreated subjects, the treated groups showed reduced bone loss. This was approximately one-third that of the untreated subjects. Amongst untreated subjects, the rate of bone loss was maximum between 56 and 70 years of age, and thereafter slowed. This indicates that for the most effective prevention against bone loss, estrogen replacement therapy should be started soon after menopause and continued long-term[77]

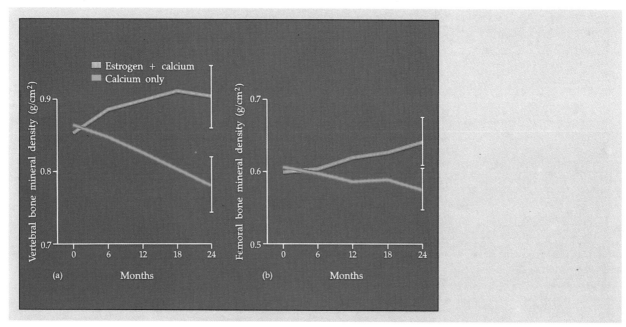

Figure 60 Effects of estrogen plus calcium compared with calcium alone on bone density in women with established osteoporosis. Forty women with vertebral crush fractures or deformities due to postmenopausal osteoporosis were randomly allocated to one of two groups. They received either conjugated equine estrogens 0.625 mg daily with calcium to achieve a calcium intake of 1500 mg/day, or calcium supplements alone during the 2-year study. A cyclical progestogen was also given to those receiving estrogen who had an intact uterus. Bone mineral density was measured in the hip and spine using DPA at 6-monthly intervals. (a) Vertebral bone density increased significantly during treatment with estrogen and calcium, whereas treatment with calcium alone led to a slow decline in bone density, although at 2 years the difference from baseline was not significant; (b) changes in the hip were similar, although they did not achieve significance in either group. Therapy with estrogen is beneficial in preventing further bone loss and even improves bone density in women with established osteoporosis. Calcium alone appears to have a less beneficial effect[78]

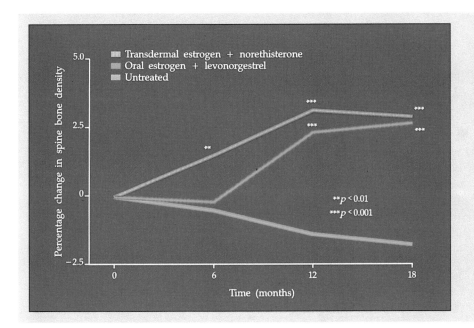

Figure 61 Comparison of oral and transdermal estrogen and progestogen therapies in preventing spinal postmenopausal bone loss. A total of 66 postmenopausal women were randomized to treatment for 18 months with either oral estrogen and progestogen (conjugated equine estrogens 0.625 mg/day with 150 µg/day dl norgestrel for 12 days of each 28-day cycle) or transdermal therapy (17β-estradiol 50 µg/day with transdermal norethisterone acetate 250 µg/day for 14 days per 28-day cycle). All women underwent assessments of spinal bone density at 6-monthly intervals. A third, matched group of 33 untreated women also underwent regular bone density assessments for comparison. At 18 months, the oral and transdermal groups showed similar bone preservation which was significantly different as compared to the loss seen in the untreated group[79]

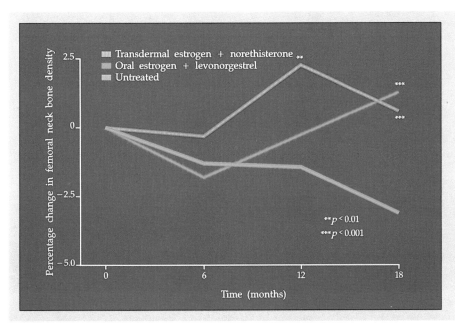

Figure 62 Percentage change in femoral neck bone density in 66 postmenopausal women randomized to treatment for 18 months with either oral estrogen and progestogen (conjugated equine estrogens 0.625 mg/day with 150 µg/day dl norgestrel for 12 days of each 28-day cycle) or transdermal therapy (17β-estradiol 50 µg/day with transdermal norethisterone acetate 250 µg/day for 14 days per 28-day cycle). A third, matched group of 33 untreated women also underwent regular (6-monthly) bone density assessments for comparison. At 18 months, bone density was significantly higher in both treatment groups as compared to that of the untreated group. These results and those in Figure 61 indicate that transdermal estrogens are as effective as oral in preventing postmenopausal bone loss in both hip and spine[79]

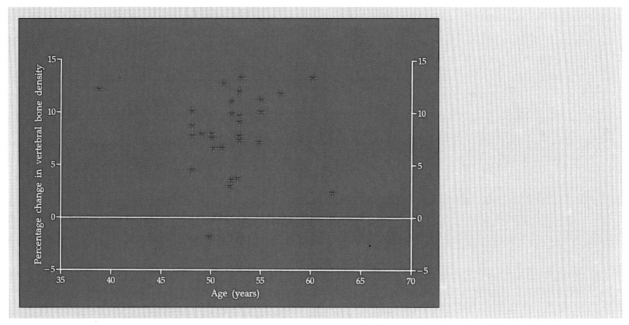

Figure 63 Effect of estradiol and testosterone implants on bone mineral density in postmenopausal women. Postmenopausal women received subcutaneous estradiol 75 mg and testosterone 100 mg implants at 6-monthly intervals for 1 year. Bone density in the vertebral spine and the femoral neck and serum estradiol levels were measured before and after 1 year. There was a significant increase in bone density in the spine (illustrated here) and in the femoral neck, and this was correlated with the rise in serum estradiol[80]

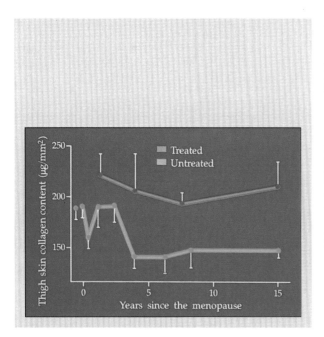

Figure 64 The effect of treatment with subcutaneous estradiol implants on thigh skin collagen in 59 postmenopausal women compared to 148 untreated women. Treatment was given for between 2 and 10 years. This figure indicates that, with estrogen replacement, thigh skin collagen content is maintained[5]

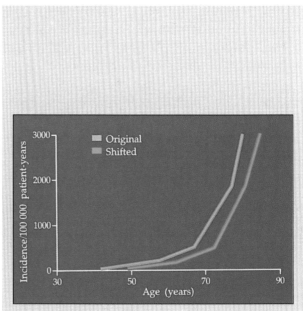

Figure 65 Effect of delaying bone loss by 5 years on fracture rate of the proximal femur. Original: age-specific incidence of fracture amongst women from Rochester, Minnesota, USA. Shifted: age-specific incidence of same population as it might appear if osteoporosis onset was delayed by 5 years. This would lead to a reduction in fracture rate of approximately 50% at any age in the population at risk, and suggests that treatment with estrogen replacement, even in the relatively short-term, has a long-term, beneficial, carry-over effect[25]

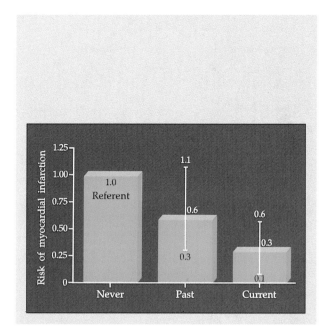

Figure 66 Effects of current, past and never use estrogen replacement therapy on risk of myocardial infarction. As part of the Nurses Health Study, 32 317 women without previous coronary heart disease completed a questionnaire providing information on their coronary risk factors and use of estrogen replacement therapy. Questionnaires were completed 3 years and 5 years later. As compared to non-users of estrogen replacement (relative risk standardized to 1.0), past users had a relative risk of 0.6 which was not significantly different to non-users (95% confidence interval [CI] 0.3–1.1). Current users, however, had a relative risk of 0.3 (95% CI 0.1–0.6) which was significantly lower than never users. In this study, the pattern of coronary risk factors (hypercholesterolemia, family history of heart disease, hypertension, diabetes, obesity and smoking, etc.) within the groups was almost identical. Thus, it is most unlikely that inclusion or selection bias is the explanation for these results. No effect of dose and duration of estrogen therapy was seen[81]

| | Estrogen replacement therapy | | | |
| | Never-use | | Ever-use | |
Risk factor	Mortality rate per 1000 women	Number of deaths	Mortality rate per 1000 women	Number of deaths
Previous myocardial infarction/angina				
No	3.8	38	2.0	19 *
Yes	10.7	18	5.2	9
Previous hypertension				
No	3.6	24	2.0	14 *
Yes	6.4	32	3.0	14 *
Smoking				
No	4.9	39	2.0	13 *
Yes	4.7	17	4.1	15

*$p < 0.05$

Figure 67 Age-adjusted mortality rates for acute myocardial infarction per 1000 women, and number of deaths by other cardiovascular risk factors and by use of estrogen replacement therapy. Females living in a retirement community in Southern California were followed over a 5-year period. Deaths from myocardial infarction were recorded. The table compares rates in users and non-users of estrogen replacement after stratifying for cardiovascular risk factors. The results show an approximate 50% reduction in deaths from myocardial infarction with estrogen use even in women with risk factors for cardiovascular disease, such as previous myocardial infarction, angina or hypertension. The one exception is cigarette smoking where use of HRT was not protective. These data again indicate that the protective effects of HRT against cardiovascular disease cannot be explained by inclusion bias, with only women at low risk for cardiovascular disease receiving treatment. Protective effects were observed in this study in 'high-risk' women[82]

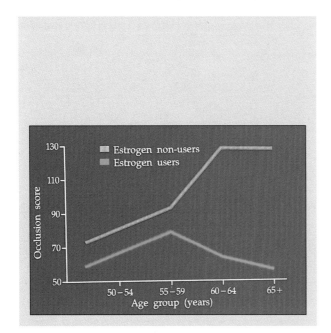

Figure 68 Coronary artery occlusion scores in users as compared to non-users of estrogen replacement therapy. Coronary occlusion scores were derived in postmenopausal women who had undergone angiography for ischemic heart disease. The relative risk in non-users was standardized to 1.0. The relative risk for current estrogen users with severe coronary occlusion was 0.37 and for those with moderate occlusion it was 0.59. This illustrates the protective effect of estrogen against further coronary occlusion, especially in those with severe occlusive disease[83]

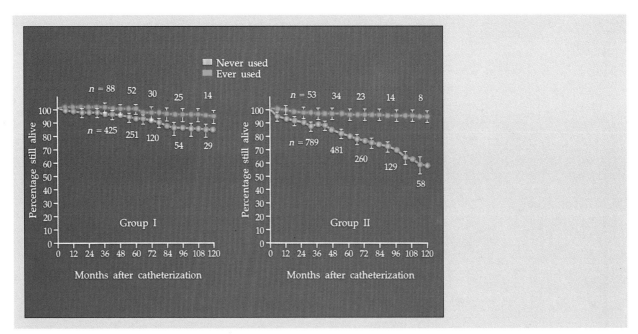

Figure 69 Effects of estrogen replacement on the 10-year survival of postmenopausal women with angiographically proven coronary artery disease. A total of 644 women had moderate disease (< 75% stenosis of one or more coronary arteries) (Group 1). Group 2 consisted of 1178 women with ≥ 70% stenosis of one or more coronary arteries or ≥ 50% reduction in the diameter of the lumen of the left main coronary artery. A group with no stenosis was recruited as control. Estrogen use was ascertained from questionnaires sent annually to patients and/or physicians. In Group 1 there was a 5-year survival of 98% in users of estrogen and 91% in non-users. At 10 years the survival was 96% in users and 85% in non-users; this difference was significant. In Group 2 the 5-year survival was 97% in users of estrogen and 81% in non-users. At 10 years, the survival remained at 97% in users and had fallen to 60% in non-users; this difference was highly significant. Estrogen treatment improves survival in women with moderate or severe coronary heart disease. This benefit appears more pronounced the greater the degree of coronary artery occlusion[84]

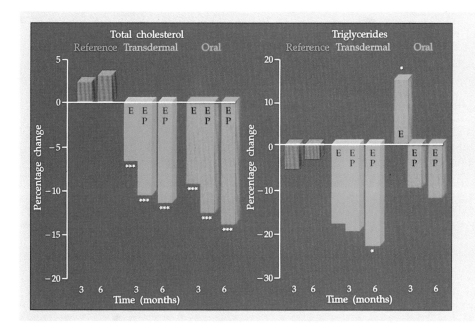

Figure 70 Comparison of the effects of oral and transdermal estrogen/progestogen on total cholesterol and serum triglycerides. Apparently healthy postmenopausal women ($n = 66$) were randomized to receive either oral estrogen and progestogen (conjugated equine estrogens 0.625 mg/ day for 28 days with dl norgestrel 150 μg/day for the last 12 days) or transdermal therapy (17β-estradiol 50 μg/day for 28 days with norethisterone acetate 250 μg/day for the last 14 days). Measurements were performed pretreatment, during the estrogen-alone (E) phase of cycle 3, and during the combined estrogen/progestogen (E + P) phases of cycles 3 and 6. An untreated group of women were studied concurrently on three occasions, 3 months apart. For all groups, the results are presented as mean percentage change from baseline. Both therapies significantly reduced total cholesterol with no differences between treatments. Transdermal therapy lowered and oral estrogen alone elevated serum triglycerides. Addition of oral progestogen was potentially advantageous and reduced triglyceride concentrations. *$p < 0.05$; ***$p < 0.001$[29]

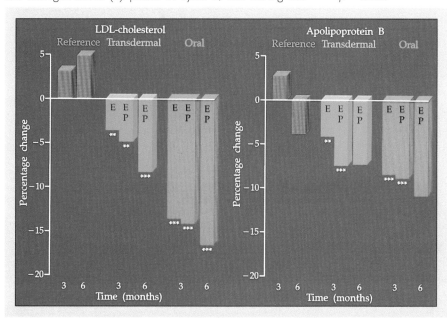

Figure 71 Comparison of the effects of oral and transdermal estrogen/progestogen on low density lipoprotein (LDL)-cholesterol and apolipoprotein B. Details of the patients, methods and expression of results are as given in the legend to Figure 70. LDL-cholesterol was significantly reduced by both therapies. There were no significant differences between treatments. In both treatment groups, the LDL levels remained low when the progestogen was added. Apolipoprotein B is the principal protein component of LDL. Changes in apolipoprotein B in this study reflected changes in LDL. **$p < 0.01$; ***$p < 0.001$[29]

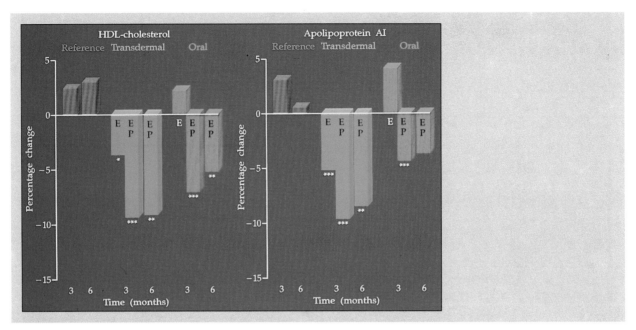

Figure 72 Comparison of the effects of oral and transdermal estrogen/progestogen on high density lipoprotein (HDL)-cholesterol and apolipoprotein AI. Details of the patients, methods and expression of results are as given in the legend to Figure 70. HDL-cholesterol was significantly reduced by both therapies in the combined phase of treatment. The elevation in HDL-cholesterol during the estrogen-only phase of cycle 3 was not significant. Apolipoprotein AI is the principal protein component of HDL. Changes in apolipoprotein AI in this study reflected changes in HDL. $*p < 0.05$; $**p < 0.01$; $***p < 0.001$[29]

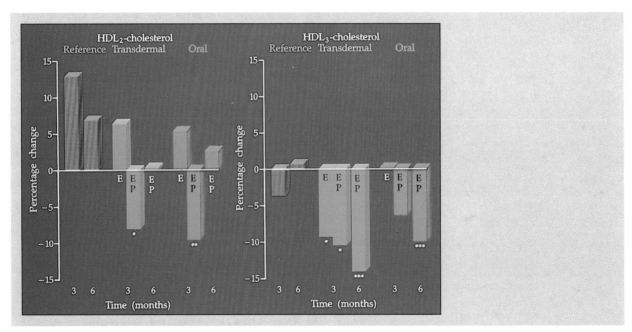

Figure 73 Comparison of the effects of oral and transdermal estrogen/progestogen on HDL_2-cholesterol and HDL_3-cholesterol. Details of the patients, methods and expression of results are as given in the legend to Figure 70. $*p < 0.05$; $**p < 0.01$; $***p < 0.001$[29]

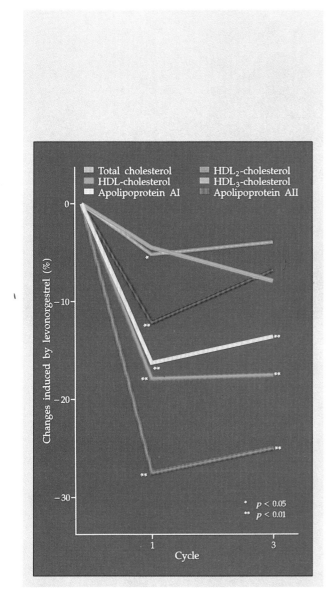

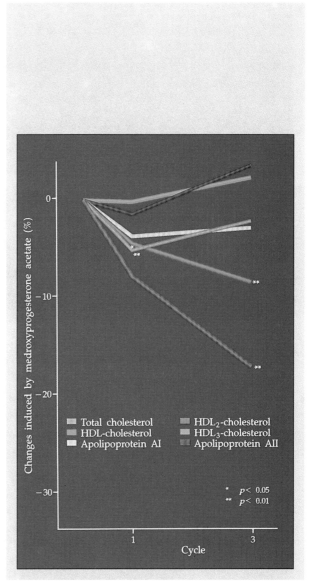

Figure 74 Effects of different progestogens on various lipids and lipoproteins. Postmenopausal women receiving oral estradiol valerate, 2 mg/day, added in levonorgestrel, 250 μg/day, for the last 12 days of each treatment cycle. The addition of this progestogen resulted in significant reductions in both HDL-cholesterol (18%) and HDL_2-cholesterol (28%). Similar changes in apolipoprotein A were observed[85]

Figure 75 Effects of different progestogens on various lipids and lipoproteins. Postmenopausal women receiving oral estradiol valerate, 2 mg/day, added in medroxyprogesterone acetate, 10 mg/day, for the last 12 days of each treatment cycle. The addition of this progestogen resulted in significant reductions in both HDL-cholesterol (8%) and HDL_2-cholesterol (17%). There were no corresponding changes in the relevant apolipoprotein fractions. These data illustrate that C-21 derivatives (such as medroxyprogesterone acetate) can cause similar lipid effects as compared to C-19 nortestosterone derivatives (e.g. levonorgestrel) (Figure 74)[85]

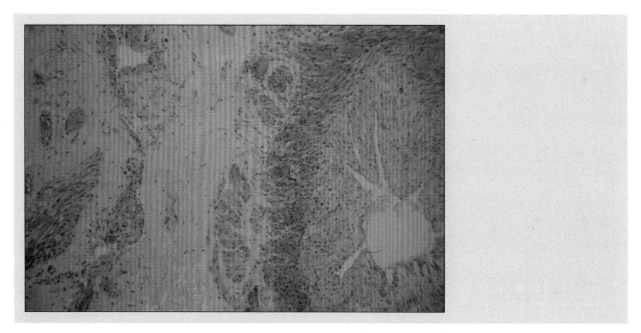

Figure 76 Staining of the muscularis of premenopausal uterine artery for the presence of a protein related to the estradiol receptor. The dense brown staining represents conversion of diamino benzidine (DAB) to an insoluble brown pigment. To assess identification of histological features, the section has been lightly counterstained with hematoxylin

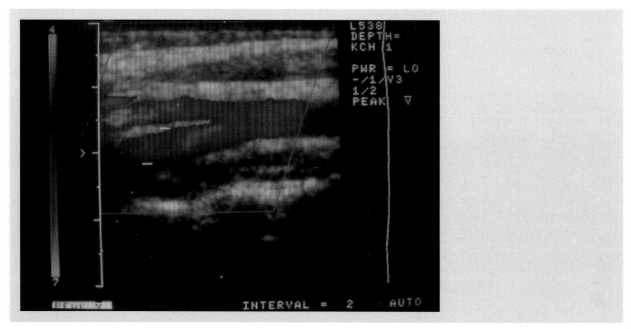

Figure 77 Doppler ultrasound scan with color flow imaging across the external and internal carotid arteries during systole. Continuous monitoring during successive cardiac cycles permits recording of the flow velocity waveform[18]

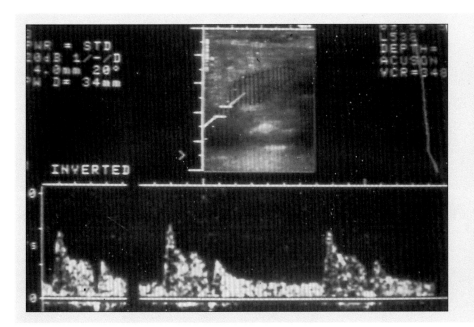

Figure 78 Flow velocity waveforms in successive cardiac cycles from a postmenopausal woman who had not taken hormone replacement therapy. Color flow imaging ('Acuson 128', Acuson, Mountain View, California) with a 5 MHz linear transducer was used to identify the common carotid artery, carotid bulb and internal and external carotid arteries. The pulsed Doppler range gate was placed across the internal carotid artery 1.5 cm distal to the carotid bifurcation (upper) to obtain flow velocity waveforms (lower)[18]

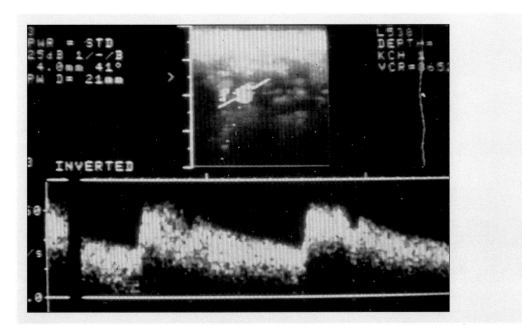

Figure 79 Flow velocity waveforms during successive cardiac cycles from the same postmenopausal woman as in Figure 78 after treatment with transdermal estradiol (Estraderm 50, Ciba-Geigy) 50 µg/day. The changes in the flow velocity waveform induced by exogenous estrogen therapy are clearly illustrated. These represent a reduction in the impedance to flow of approximately 30%[18]

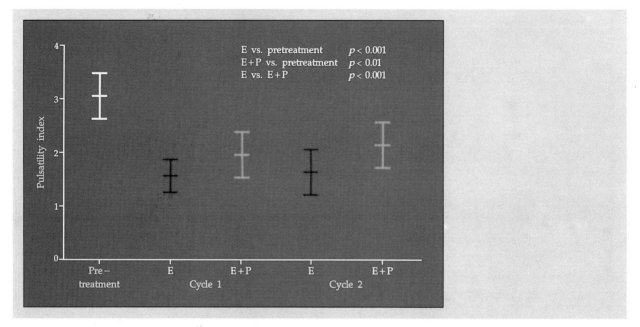

Figure 80 Flow velocity waveforms were obtained from the uterine arteries of 12 postmenopausal women pretreatment and during the estrogen-only (E) and estrogen/progestogen (E + P) phases of treatment over the next 2 months. From the flow velocity waveforms, the pulsatility index (PI) of the uterine arteries was calculated. The PI is believed to represent impedance to flow downstream from the point of sampling. Mean (95% confidence interval) values for uterine artery pulsatility index before and then during treatment are as shown[86]

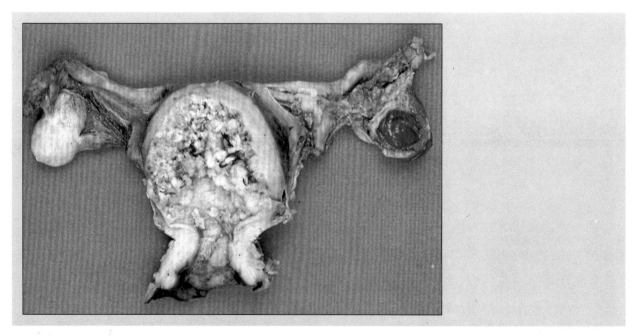

Figure 81 Endometrial carcinoma. The incidence of this disease is approximately 1 per 1000 women per annum between the ages of 50 and 60 years. This is the most common gynecological malignancy in postmenopausal women, even without the use of unopposed estrogens. It usually presents with postmenopausal bleeding. Any episode of postmenopausal bleeding, therefore, demands endometrial assessment

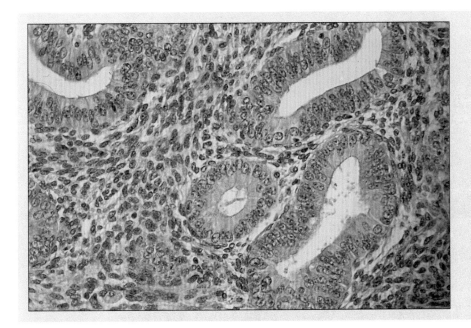

Figure 82 Endometrial carcinoma is characterized by large pleomorphic cells with loss of polarity and atypical nuclei with many mitoses. Hemotoxylin and eosin: magnification × 250

	Number of cases observed	Number of cases expected	Relative risk	95% confidence intervals
Estradiol	30	14.4	2.1	1.4 – 3.0
Conjugated estrogens	21	12.3	1.7	1.1 – 2.7
Other estrogens	19	20.8	0.9	0.6 – 1.4

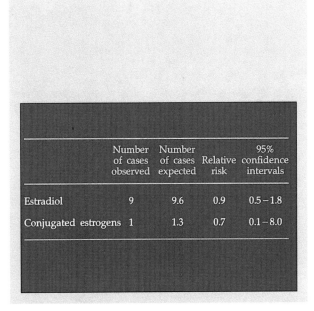

	Number of cases observed	Number of cases expected	Relative risk	95% confidence intervals
Estradiol	9	9.6	0.9	0.5 – 1.8
Conjugated estrogens	1	1.3	0.7	0.1 – 8.0

Figure 83 Effects of exogenous estrogen therapy (not opposed by a progestogen) on the relative risk of endometrial neoplasia (hyperplasia plus carcinoma). Altogether 23 244 women were followed for 6 years in a prospective population-based study. Their use of hormone replacement therapy was recorded and this included details of type and duration of treatment. All new cases of endometrial hyperplasia and carcinoma were obtained from the National Cancer Registry. The relative risks (95% confidence intervals) are shown related to duration of therapy (months)[33]

Figure 84 Effects of exogenous estrogen/progestogen therapy on the relative risk of endometrial neoplasia (hyperplasia plus carcinoma). A total of 23 244 women were followed for 6 years in a prospective population-based study. Their use of hormone replacement therapy was recorded and this included details of type and duration of treatment. All new cases of endometrial hyperplasia and carcinoma were obtained from the National Cancer Registry. The relative risks (95% confidence intervals) as shown related to duration of therapy (months)[33]

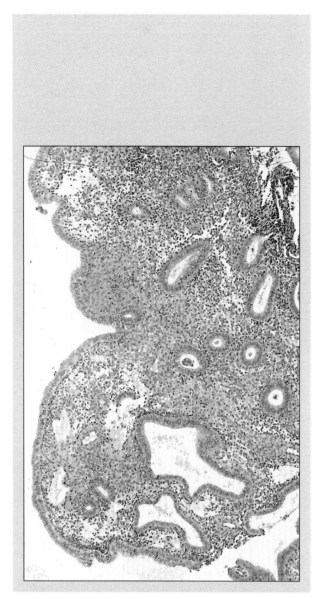

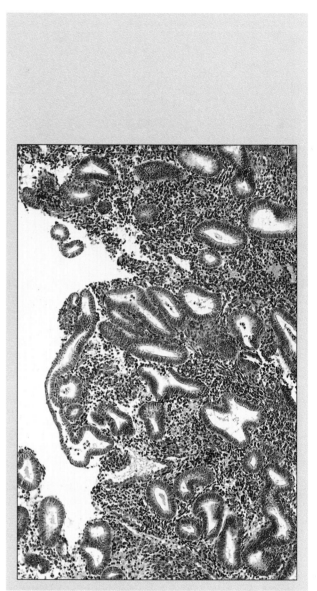

Figure 85 Cystic hyperplasia of the endometrium. This condition results from prolonged estrogenic stimulation not opposed by progesterone/progestogen. It occurs most commonly with perimenopausal anovulatory cycles or with exogenous estrogen administered without progestogen. Histologically, there is a loss of distinction between the basal and superficial layers of the endometrium. The cells are crowded, with increased mitosis being present in the glands and stroma. The glands are straight and cylindrical, and are lined with columnar cells with a basophilic cytoplasm. If left untreated, approximately 1–2% of cystic hyperplasias are believed to progress to malignancy

Figure 86 Atypical hyperplasia of the endometrium. This is characterized by gland crowding with 'back-to-back' gland formation, proliferation of the cells ('tufting') lining the glands, and by many and abnormal mitoses. In severe cases, differentiation between atypical hyperplasia and well differentiated adenocarcinoma can be difficult. It has been suggested that the risk of subsequent malignant change is related to the severity of the atypical hyperplasia. Thus, mild forms may carry a risk of subsequent malignant change of around 12–15%. This is increased to 25% with moderate atypical hyperplasia, and to 50% or more with the most severe forms

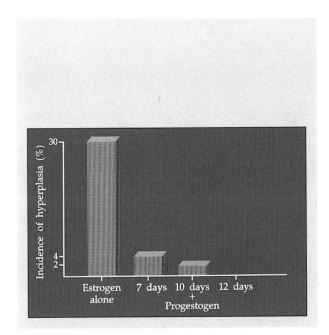

Figure 87 Incidence of hyperplasia in postmenopausal women receiving unopposed estrogens or estrogen with a progestogen added for the stated number of days each cycle/calendar month. Estrogens unopposed by a progestogen are associated with a 20–30% incidence of hyperplasia over approximately 18 months. The addition of a progestogen for 7 days reduced the incidence to 4%, for 10 days to 2%, and for 12 days to zero. Duration of progestogen administration appears to be as important as daily dosage in reducing the risk of endometrial hyperplasia[87]

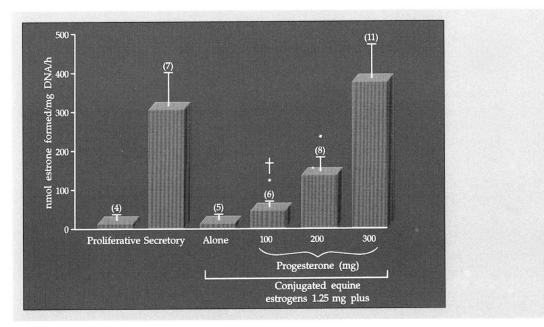

Figure 88 Activity of 17β-estradiol dehydrogenases in the endometrium of postmenopausal women treated with conjugated equine estrogens 1.25 mg/day continuously, either alone or with oral natural progesterone 100 mg, 200 mg, or 300 mg daily added for 10 days each calendar month. Proliferative and secretory phase ranges are included for comparison. Results are expressed as means (SEM). The numbers of observations are given in parentheses. p values (Student's t-test) represent the following significant differences: conjugated estrogens alone versus conjugated estrogens plus progesterone: $*p < 0.001$; conjugated estrogens plus progesterone versus premenopausal secretory phase: $†p < 0.001$[88]

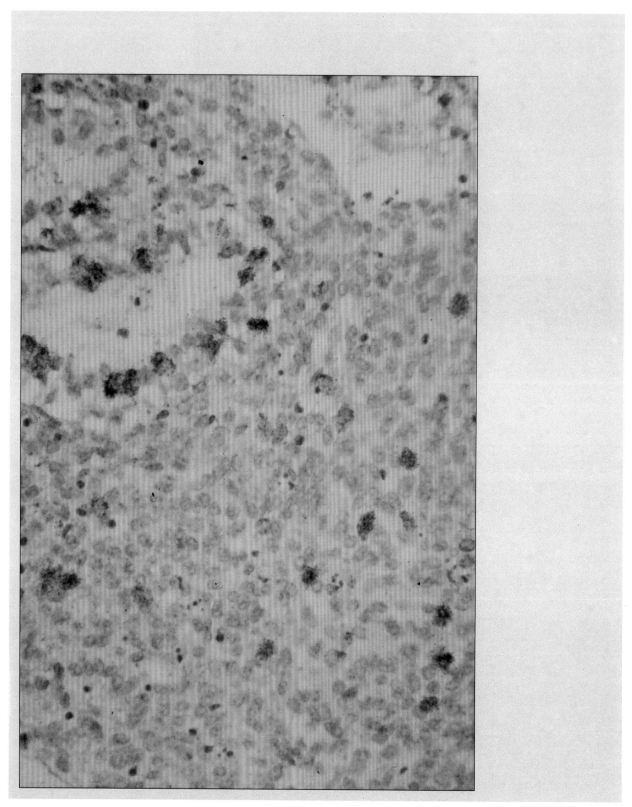

Figure 89 Autoradiogram prepared from a postmenopausal endometrium after incubation with tritiated thymidine. The labelled cells in both epithelium and stroma are shown clearly[89]

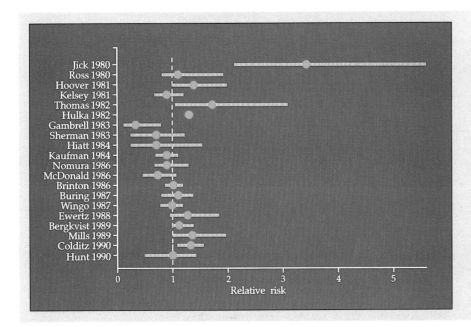

Figure 90 Summary of epidemiological studies[32,36-39,41-47,90-96] which have reported the relative risk of breast cancer in HRT users. Results are shown as relative risk with confidence intervals. Numerous workers have investigated this relationship during the last 10 years and the results of 21 such studies are sum-marized here. The risk of breast cancer in non-users of HRT has been standardized to 1.0. With the exception of the results of Jick et al. (1980), most studies report a modest increase or a slight decrease in risk.

The lack of consensus as to the true effects of HRT on breast cancer risk makes it very difficult for the physician to counsel women requesting information about use of HRT and risk of breast cancer. This summary shows the *overall* relative risk reported by each of these studies. The overall relative risk takes no account of factors such as duration of therapy and presence of pre-existing breast disease which may influence risk (see Figures 91 and 93)

Years of use	Cases	Controls	Relative risk	95% confidence intervals
<5	486	640	0.89	0.8–1.0
5–9	249	259	1.09	0.9–1.3
10–14	159	141	1.28	0.9–1.6
15–19	70	74	1.24	0.9–1.8
20+	49	43	1.47	0.9–2.3
Trend test	6.31 ($p < 0.01$)			

Figure 91 Effect of duration of use of postmenopausal estrogen therapy on relative risk of breast carcinoma. A total of 1960 postmenopausal women with breast carcinoma were identified from a breast cancer screening program and their history of estrogen use was recorded. Increasing duration of use appeared to be associated with an increase in risk. However, none of the increased relative risks, even that of 1.47 with 20 or more years use of HRT, achieved statistical significance. The trend test for the increases in relative risk with time was significant ($p < 0.01$). The increases in risk observed with extended durations of use applied to all subgroups of women, including those who had undergone oophorectomy and those who had undergone natural menopause[38]

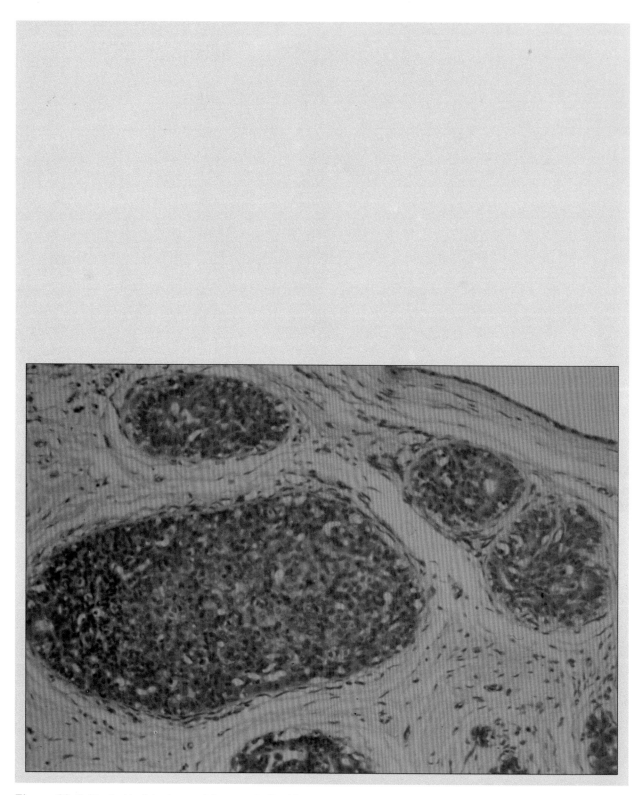

Figure 92 Epitheliosis of the breast. Microscopically, this is characterized by hyperplasia of the epithelium lining the ducts and acini. This leads to the ducts and acini eventually becoming filled with hyperplastic epithelial cells. This condition appears to be associated with an increase in life-time risk of breast carcinoma, particularly when the cells exhibit atypical change and/or the presence of calcification

History of biopsy for benign breast disease and timing of hormone use	Cases	Controls	Relative risk	95% confidence intervals
Biopsy, no hormone use	190	167	1.00	–
Hormone use before first biopsy				
ever use	48	70	0.60	0.4 – 0.9
< 10 years use	29	40	0.62	0.4 – 1.1
10+ years use	19	30	0.62	0.3 – 1.2
Hormone use after first biopsy				
ever use	205	152	1.14	0.8 – 1.6
< 10 years use	148	134	0.93	0.7 – 1.3
10+ years use	57	18	3.01	1.6 – 5.5

Figure 93 Relative risk (95% confidence intervals) of breast cancer related to history of benign breast disease and timing of postmenopausal estrogen use. Postmenopausal women developing benign breast disease *after* starting HRT had an overall relative risk for breast cancer of 0.60 (0.4–0.9, 95% confidence intervals). This was not influenced by duration of use of HRT. Women with a history of benign breast disease who subsequently used HRT for less than 10 years were not at an increase in risk of breast cancer (relative risk 0.93, 95% confidence intervals 0.7–1.3). However, if the duration of use of HRT was 10 years or more, then such women were at a significantly increased risk for breast cancer (relative risk 3.01, 95% confidence intervals 1.6–5.5). These data suggest that the increase in risk conferred by benign breast disease is further enhanced by long-term use of estrogen. However, it is not clear whether the relative risk of 3.01 in long-term users of HRT is due entirely to the natural expression of benign breast disease, or is due in part to this plus use of estrogens. Women in this study developing benign breast disease after starting HRT were not at an increase in risk of breast cancer, even with long-term use of estrogens[38]

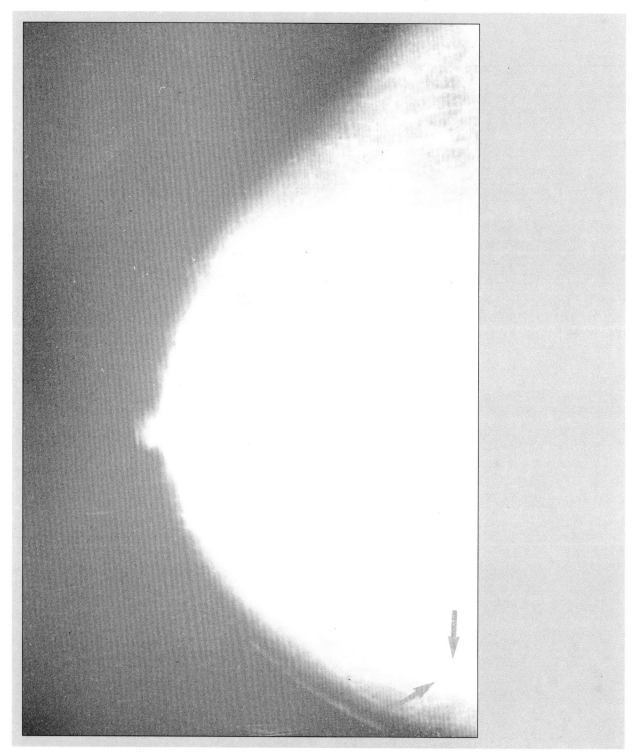

Figure 94 Mammogram of 7 mm invasive carcinoma in a 51-year old woman. The Forrest Report concluded that single mediolateral oblique view mammography is effective in reducing mortality from breast carcinoma. The report also concluded that regular screening may reduce breast cancer mortality

Acknowledgements *to the original sources of the referenced illustrations in Section 2*

The following figures have been *adapted* from the sources listed below by kind permission of the publishers and, where relevant, the authors.

Figure 1 Cope, E. (1976). Physical changes associated with the post-menopausal years. In Campbell, S. (ed.) *The Management of the Menopause and Postmenopausal Years.* p. 33. (Lancaster: MTP Press)

Figure 3 Speroff, L., Glass, R. and Case, N. (1983). *Clinical Gynecological Endocrinology and Infertility.* (Baltimore: Williams and Wilkins)

Figure 4 Whitehead, M. and Studd, J. W. W. (1988). Selection of patients for treatment. Which therapy and for how long? In Studd, J. W. W. and Whitehead, M. I. (eds.) *The Menopause,* p. 117. (Oxford: Blackwell Scientific)

Figures 5 and 6 Sturdee, D. *Modern Medicine of Great Britain*

Figure 7 Molnar, G. W. (1975). Body temperatures during menopausal hot flushes. *J. Appl. Physiol.,* **38**, 499–503

Figure 8 Bungay, G. T., Vessey, M. P. and McPherson, C. K. (1980). Study of symptoms in middle life with especial reference to the menopause. *Br. Med. J.,* **2**, 181–3

Figures 11 and 13 Dempster, D., Shane, E., Horbert, W. and Lindsay, R. (1986). A simple method for correlative scanning electron microscopy of human iliac crest biopsies. *Am. J. Bone Min. Res.,* **1**, 15–21

Figure 27 Gordon, T., Kannel, W. B., Hjortland, M. C. and MacNamara, P. M. (1978). Menopause and coronary heart disease: the Framingham study. *Ann. Intern. Med.,* 89, 157–61

Figure 28 Colditz, G. A., Willett, W. C., Stampfer, M. J., Rosner, B., Speizer, F. E. and Hennekens, C. H. (1987). Menopause and the risk of coronary heart disease in women. *N. Engl. J. Med.,* **316**, 1105–10

Figures 29, 30, 31, 32 and 33 Stevenson, J. C., Crook, D. and Godsland, I. F. (1993). Influence of age and menopause on serum lipids and lipoproteins in healthy women. *Atherosclerosis,* **98**, 83–90

Figure 36 Gambrell, R. D. Jr. (1983). Breast disease in the postmenopausal years. *Sem. Reprod. Endocrinol.,* **1**, 27–40

Figure 39 Key, T. J. and Pike, M. C. (1988). The role of oestrogens and progestogens in the epidemiology and prevention of breast carcinoma. *Eur. J. Cancer Clin. Oncol.,* **24**, 29–43

Figure 40 Mashchak, C. A., Lobo, R. A., Dozono-Takano, R., Eggena, P., Nakamura, R. M., Brenner, P. F. and Mischell, D. R. (1982). Comparison of pharmacodynamic properties of various estrogen formulations. *Am. J. Obstet. Gynecol.,* **144**, 511–18

Figure 43 Barlow, D. H., Abdullah, H. I., Roberts, A. D., Al-Azzawi, F., Leggate, I. and Hart, D. M. (1986). Long-term hormone implant therapy – hormonal and clinical effects. *Obstet. Gynecol.,* **67**, 321–5
and
Whitehead, M. and Godfree, V. (1992). *Hormone Replacement Therapy: Your Questions Answered,* p. 99. (Edinburgh: Churchill Livingstone)

Figure 44 Jensen, J. and Christiansen, C. (1983). Dose response and withdrawal effects of climacteric symptoms after hormonal replacement therapy. A placebo-controlled therapeutic trial. *Maturitas,* **5**, 125–33

Figures 45, 46 and 47 Campbell, S. and Whitehead, M. I. (1977). Oestrogen therapy and the menopausal syndrome. In

Greenblatt, R. B. and Studd, J. W. W. (eds.) *Clinics in Obstetrics and Gynecology*, Vol. 4, no. 1, pp. 31–47. (Philadelphia: W. B. Saunders)

Figure 49 Padwick, M. L. Endacott, J. and Whitehead, M. I. (1985). Efficacy, acceptability and metabolic effects of transdermal estradiol in the management of postmenopausal women. *Am. J. Obstet. Gynecol.*, **152**, 1085–91

Figures 50 and 51 Schiff, I. Tulchinsky, D. and Ryan, K. J. (1977). Vaginal absorption of oestrone and oestradiol 17-β. *Fertil. Steril.*, **28**, 1063

Figure 52 Dyer, G. I., Young, O., Townsend, P. T., Collins, W. P. and Whitehead, M. I. (1982). Dose-related changes in vaginal cytology after topical conjugated equine oestrogens. *Br. Med. J.*, **284**, 789

Figure 53 Cardozo, L. D., Gibb, D. M. F., Studd, J. W. W., Tuck, S. M., Thom, M. H. and Cooper, D. J. (1983). The effects of subcutaneous hormone implant during the climacteric. *Maturitas*, **5**, 177–84

Figure 54 Brincat, M., Studd, J., O'Dowd, T., Magos, A., Cardozo, L. D., Wardle, P. J. and Cooper, D. (1984). Subcutaneous hormone implants for the control of climacteric symptoms. *Lancet*, **I**, 16–18

Figures 55, 56 and 57 Fraser, D., Padwick, M. L., Whitehead, M. I., Coffer, A. and King, R. J. B. (1991). Presence of an oestradiol receptor-related protein in the skin: changes during the normal menstrual cycle. *Br. J. Obstet. Gynecol.*, **98**, 1277–82

Figure 58 Melton, J., Wahner, H., Richelson, L., O'Fallon, M. and Riggs, B. (1986). Osteoporosis and the risk of hip fracture. *Am. J. Epidemiol.*, **124**, 254–61

Figure 59 Quigley, M., Purvis, L., Martin, M., Burnier, A. and Brooks, P. (1987). Estrogen therapy arrests bone loss in elderly women. *Am. J. Obstet. Gynecol.*, **156**, 1516–21

Figure 60 Lindsay, R. and Tohme, J. (1990). Estrogen treatment of patients with established postmenopausal osteoporosis. *Obstet. Gynecol.*, **76**, 290–5

Figures 61 and 62 Stevenson, J. C., Cust, M., Gangar, K. F., Hillard, T. C., Lees, B. and Whitehead, M. I. (1990). Effects of transdermal versus oral hormone replacement therapy on bone density in the spine and proximal femur of postmenopausal women. *Lancet*, **335**, 265–9

Figure 63 Studd, J., Savvas, M., Watson, N., Garnett, T., Fogelman, I. and Cooper, D. (1990). The relationship between plasma oestradiol and the increase in bone density in the postmenopausal women after treatment with subcutaneous implants. *Am. J. Obstet. Gynecol.*, **163**, 474–9

Figure 64 Brincat, M., Moniz, C. J., Studd, J. W. W., Darby,

A., Magos, A., Emburey, G. and Versi, E. (1985). Long-term effects of the menopause and sex hormones on skin thickness. *Br. J. Obstet. Gynaecol.*, **92**, 256–9

Figure 65 Melton, L. J. (1987). Postmenopausal bone loss and osteoporosis: epidemiological aspects. In Zichella, L., Whitehead, M. I. and Van Keep, P. A. (eds.) *The Climacteric and Beyond*, pp. 127–9. (Carnforth, UK: Parthenon Publishing)

Figure 66 Stampfer, M. J., Willett, W. C., Colditz, G. A., Rosner, B., Speizer, F. E. and Hennekens, C. H. (1985). A prospective study of postmenopausal estrogen therapy and coronary heart disease. *N. Engl. J. Med.*, **313**, 1044–9

Figure 67 Henderson, B. E., Ross, R. K., Paganini-Hill, A. and Mack, T. M. (1986). Estrogen use and cardiovascular disease. *Am. J. Obstet. Gynecol.*, **154**, 1181–6

Figure 68 Gruchow, H. W., Anderson, A. J., Barboriak, J. J. and Sobocinski, K. A. (1988). Postmenopausal use of estrogen and occlusion of coronary arteries. *Am. Heart J.*, **115**, 954–63

Figure 69 Sullivan, J. M., Van der Zwagg, R., Hughes, J. P., Maddock, V., Kroetz, F. W., Ramanathan, K. B. and Mirvis, D. M. (1990). Estrogen replacement and coronary artery disease – effect on survival in postmenopausal women. *Arch. Intern. Med.*, **150**, 2557–62

Figures 70, 71, 72 and 73 Crook, D., Cust, M., Gangar, K., Worthington, M., Hillard, T., Stevenson, J. C., Whitehead, M. I. and Wynn, V. (1992). Comparison of transdermal and oral estrogen/progestin replacement therapy: effects on serum lipids and lipoproteins. *Am. J. Obstet. Gynecol.*, **166**, 950–5

Figures 74 and 75 Ottoson, U. B., Johansson, B. G. and von Schoultz, B. (1985). Subfractions of high-density lipoprotein cholesterol during estrogen replacement therapy: a comparison between progestogens and natural progesterone. *Am. J. Obstet. Gynecol.*, **151**, 746–50

Figures 77, 78 and 79 Gangar, K., Vyas, S., Whitehead, M. I., Crook, D., Meire, H. and Campbell, S. (1991). Pulsatility index in internal carotid artery in relation to transdermal oestradiol and time since menopause. *Lancet*, **338**, 839–42

Figure 80 Hillard, T. C., Bourne, T. H., Whitehead, M. I., Crayford, T. B., Collins, W. P. and Campbell, S. (1992). Differential effects of transdermal estradiol and sequential progestogens on impedance to flow within the uterine arteries of postmenopausal women. *Fertil. Steril.*, **58**, 959–63

Figures 83 and 84 Persson, I., Adami, H. A., Bergkvist, L., Lindgren, A., Pettersson, B., Hoover, R. and Schairer, C. (1989). Risk of endometrial cancer after treatment with oestrogens alone or in conjunction with progestogens: results of a prospective study. *Br. Med. J.*, **298**, 147–51

Figure 87 Whitehead, M. I., Hillard, T. C. and Crook, D. (1990). The role and use of progestogens. *Obstet. Gynecol.*, **75**, 59–76S

Figure 88 Lane, G., Siddle, N. C., Ryder, T. A., Pryse-Davis, J., King, R. J. B. and Whitehead, M. I. (1983). Dose dependent effects or oral progesterone on the oestrogenised postmenopausal endometrium. *Br. Med. J.*, **287**, 1241–5

Figure 89 Whitehead, M. I., Townsend, P. T., Pryse-Davis, J., Ryder, T., Lane, G., Siddle, N. C. and King, R. J. B. (1982). Effects of various types and dosages of progestogens on the postmenopausal endometrium. *J. Reprod. Med.*, **27**, 539–48

Figures 91 and 93 Brinton, L. A., Hoover, R. and Fraumeni, J. F. (1986). Menopausal oestrogens and breast cancer risk: an expanded case-control study. *Br. J. Cancer*, **54**, 825–32

Figures 19, 38, 81, 82, 92 and 94 are reproduced by kind permission of the Graves National Medical Library.
Figures 20, 22, 23, 24 and 37 are reproduced by kind permission of St. Bartholomew's Hospital Medical School.
Figure 76 is reproduced by courtesy of Drs Malcolm Padwick and David Fraser of the Menopause Clinic at King's College Hospital and of Drs Arnold Coffer and Roger King of the Hormone Biochemistry Department at the Imperial Cancer Research Fund Laboratories, London.
Figure 90 is reproduced by permission of Dr Valerie Godfree of the Amarant Clinic, London. Data were compiled from references 32, 36–39, 41–47, 63, 90–96.

Section 3 Bibliography

1. Nesheim, B. I. and Saetre, T. (1982). Changes in skin blood flow and body temperatures during climacteric hot flushes. *Maturitas*, **4**, 4–55

2. Erlik, Y., Tataryn, I. V., Meldrum, D. R., Lomax, P., Bajorek, J. G. and Judd, H. L. (1981). Association of wakening episodes with menopausal hot flushes. *J. Am. Med. Assoc.*, **245**, 1741–7

3. Bungay, G. T., Vessey, M. P. and McPherson, C. K. (1980). Study of symptoms in middle life with especial reference to the menopause. *Br. Med. J.*, **2**, 181–3

4. Stumpf, W. E., Sur, M. and Joshi, S. E. (1976). Oestrogen target cells in the skin. *Experientia*, **30**, 196

5. Brincat, M., Moniz, C. J., Studd, J. W. W., Darby, A., Magos, A., Emburey, G. and Versi, E. (1985). Long-term effects of the menopause and sex hormones on skin thickness. *Br. J. Obstet. Gynaecol.*, **92**, 256–9

6. Jensen, J., Christiansen, C. and Boesen, J. (1982). Epidemiology of postmenopausal spinal and longbone fractures: a unifying approach to postmenopausal osteoporosis. *Clin. Orthopaed. Rel. Res.*, **166**, 75–81

7. Melton, L. J. and Riggs, B. L. (1983). Epidemiology of age related fractures. In Avioli, L. L. (ed.) *The Osteoporotic Syndrome*, Vol. 298, pp. 924–8. (New York: Grune and Stratton)

8. Seeman, E., Hopper, J. L. and Bach, L. A. (1989). Reduced mass in daughters of women with osteoporosis. *N. Engl. J. Med.*, **320**, 554–8

9. Stevenson, J. C., Lees, B., Devenport, M., Cust, M. P. and Gangar, K. F. (1989). Determinants of bone density in normal women: risk factors for future osteoporosis? *Br. Med. J.*, **298**, 924–8

10. Rosenberg, L., Hennekens, C. H., Rosner, B., Belanger, C., Rothman, K. J. and Speizer, F. E. (1981). Early menopause and the risk of myocardial infarction. *Am. J. Obstet. Gynecol.*, **139**, 47–51

11. Gordon, T., Kannel, W. B., Hjortland, M. C. and MacNamara, P. M. (1978). Menopause and coronary heart disease: the Framingham study. *Ann. Intern. Med.*, **89**, 157–61

12. Paganini-Hill, A., Ross, R. K. and Henderson, B. E. (1988). Post-menopausal oestrogen treatment and stroke: a prospective study. *Br. Med. J.*, **297**, 519–22

13. Ross, R. K., Paganini-Hill, A., Mack, T. M., Arthur, M. and Henderson, B. E. (1981). Menopausal oestrogen therapy and protection from death and ischaemic heart disease. *Lancet*, **1**, 858–60

14. Bush, T. L., Barrett-Conor, E. and Cowan, L. D. (1987). Cardiovascular mortality and non-contraceptive use of oestrogen in women. Results from the Lipid Research Clinics Program follow-up Study. *Circulation*, **75**, 1102–9

15. Wahl, P., Walden, C. and Knopp, R. (1983). Effect of estrogen/progestogen potency on lipid lipoprotein cholesterol. *N. Engl. J. Med.*, **308**, 862–7

16. Padwick, M., Whitehead, M. I., Offer, A. and King, R. (1986). Demonstration of oestrogen receptor related protein in female tissues. In Studd, J. W. W. and Whitehead, M. I. (eds.) *The Menopause*, pp. 227–33. (London: Blackwell Scientific Publications)

17. Bourne, T., Hillard, T. C., Whitehead, M. I., Crook, D. and Campbell, S. (1990). Oestrogen, arterial status and postmenopausal women. *Lancet*, **1**, 1470–1

18. Gangar, K., Vyas, S., Whitehead, M. I., Crook, D., Meire, H. and Campbell, S. (1991). Pulsatility index in internal carotid artery in relation to transdermal oestradiol and time since menopause. *Lancet*, **338**, 839–42

19. Campbell, S., Beard, R. J. and McQueen, J. (1976). Double blind psychometric studies on the effects of natural oestrogens on postmenopausal women. In Campbell, S. (ed.) *The Management of the Menopause and Postmenopausal Years*, pp. 149–58. (Lancaster: MTP Press)

20. Schiff, I., Regestein, Q. and Tulchinsky, D. (1979). Effects of estrogen on sleep and the psychologic state of hypogonadal women. *J. Am. Med. Assoc.*, **242**, 2405–7

21. Versi, E. and Cardozo, L. (1986). Oestrogens and lower urinary tract function. In Studd, J. W. W. and Whitehead, M. I. (eds.) *The Menopause*, pp. 76–84. (London: Blackwell Scientific Publications)

22. Padwick, M. L., Endacott, J. and Whitehead, M. I. (1985). Efficacy, acceptability and metabolic effects of transdermal estradiol in the management of postmenopausal women. *Am. J. Obstet. Gynecol.*, **152**, 1085–91

23. Lindsay, R., Hart D. M., Aitken, J. M., MacDonald, E. B., Anson, J. B. and Clark, A. C. (1976). Long-term prevention of postmenopausal osteoporosis by oestrogen. *Lancet*, **I**, 1038–41

24. Ettinger, B., Genant, H. K. and Cann, C. E. (1985). Long-term estrogen replacement therapy prevents bone loss and fractures. *Ann. Intern. Med.*, **102**, 319–24

25. Melton, L. J. (1987). Postmenopausal bone loss and osteoporosis: epidemiological aspects. In Zichella, L., Whitehead, M. I. and Van Keep, P. A. (eds.) *The Climacteric and Beyond*, pp. 127–9. (Carnforth, UK: Parthenon Publishing)

26. MacIntyre, I., Stevenson, J. C., Whitehead, M. I., Wimalawansa, S. J., Banks, L. M. and Healy, M. J. R. (1988). *Lancet*, **I**, 900–1

27. Overgaard, K., Riis, B. J., Christiansen, C., Podenphant, J. and Johansen, J. S. (1989). Nasal calcitonin for the treatment of established osteoporosis. *Clin. Endocrinol.*, **30**, 435–42

28. Storm, T., Thamsborg, G., Steiniche, T., Genant, H. K. and Soremsen, O. H. (1990). Effect of intermittent cyclical etidronate therapy on bone mass and fracture rate in women with postmenopausal osteoporosis. *N. Engl. J. Med.*, **322**, 1265–71

29. Crook, D., Cust, M., Gangar, K., Worthington, M., Hillard, T., Stevenson, J. C., Whitehead, M. I. and Wynn, V. (1992). Comparison of transdermal and oral estrogen/progestin replacement therapy: effects on serum lipids and lipoproteins. *Am. J. Obstet. Gynecol.*, **166**, 950–5

30. Hirvonen, E., Malkonen, N. and Manninen, V. (1981). Effects of different progestogens on lipo-proteins during postmenopausal replacement therapy. *N. Engl. J. Med.*, **304**, 560–5

31. Jensen, G. F., Christiansen, C., Boesen, J., Hegedus, V. and Transbol, I. (1982). Epidemiology of post-menopausal spinal and long bone fractures: a unifying approach to post-menopausal osteoporosis. *J. Orthopaed. Res. Reg.*, **166**, 75–81

32. Hunt, K., Vessey, M. P. and McPherson, K. (1990). Mortality in a cohort of long-term users of hormone replacement therapy: an updated analysis. *Br. J. Obstet. Gynaecol.*, **97**, 1080–6

33. Persson, I., Adami, H. A., Bergkvist, L., Lindgren, A., Pettersson, B., Hoover, R. and Schairer, C. (1989). Risk of endometrial cancer after treatment with oestrogens alone or in conjunction with progestogens: results of a prospective study. *Br. Med. J.*, **298**, 147–51

34. Padwick, M. L., Pryse-Davies, J. and Whitehead, M. I. (1986). A simple method for determining the optimal dose of progestin in postmenopausal women receiving estrogens. *N. Engl. J. Med.*, **315**, 930–4

35. Christiansen, C. and Riis, B. J. (1990). Five years with continuous combined oestrogen/progestin therapy. Effects on calcium metabolism, lipids and lipo-proteins and bleeding pattern. *Br. J. Obstet. Gynaecol.*, **97**, 1087–92

36. Jick, H., Walker, A., Watkins, R., D'Ewart, D., Hunter, J., Danford, A., Madsen, S., Dinan, D. and Rothman, K. (1980). Replacement estrogens and breast cancer. *Am. J. Epidemiol.*, **112**, 586–92

37. Thomas, D. B., Persing, J. P. and Hutchinson, W. B. (1982). Exogenous estrogens and other risk factors for breast cancer in women with benign breast diseases. *J. Natl. Cancer Inst.*, **69**, 1017–23

38. Brinton, L. A., Hoover, R. and Fraumeni, J. F. (1986). Menopausal oestrogens and breast cancer risk: an expanded case-control study. *Br. J. Cancer*, **54**, 825–32

39. Hiatt, R. A., Bawol, R., Friedman, G. D. and Hoover, R. (1984). Exogenous oestrogens and breast cancer after bilateral oophorectomy. *Cancer*, **54**, 139–44

40. Dupont, W. D., Page, D. L., Rogers, L. W. and Parl, F. F. (1989). Influence of exogenous estrogens, proliferative breast

diseases and other variables on breast cancer risk. *Cancer*, **63**, 948–57

41. Ross, R. K., Paganini-Hill, A., Gerkins, V. R., Mack, T. M., Pfeffer, R., Arthur, M. and Henderson, B. E. (1980). A case control study of menopausal estrogen therapy and breast cancer. *J. Am. Med. Assoc.*, **243**, 1635–9

42. Hoover, R., Glass, A., Finkle, W. D., Azvedo, G. and Milne, K. (1981). Conjugated estrogens and breast cancer risk in women. *J. Clin. Invest.*, **67**, 815–20

43. Ewertz, M. (1988). Influence of non-contraceptive exogenous and endogenous sex hormones in breast cancer risk in Denmark. *Int. J. Cancer*, **42**, 832–8

44. Kelsey, J. L., Fischer, D. B., Holford, T. R., LiVolsi, V. A., Mostow, E. D., Goldenberg, I. S. and White, C. (1981). Exogenous estrogens and other factors in the epidemiology of breast cancer. *J. Natl. Cancer Inst.*, **67**, 327–33

45. Kaufmann, D. W., Miller, D. R., Rosenberg, L., Helmrich, S. P., Stolley, P., Schottenfeld, D. and Shapiro, S. (1984). Non-contraceptive estrogen use and the risk of breast cancer. *J. Am. Med. Assoc.*, **252**, 63–7

46. Wingo, P. A., Layde, P. M., Lee, N. C., Rubin, G. and Ory, H. W. (1987). The risk of breast cancer in post menopausal women who have used estrogen replacement therapy. *J. Am. Med. Assoc.*, **257**, 209–15

47. Colditz, G. A., Stampfer, M. J., Willett, W. C., Hennekens, C. H., Rosner, B. and Speizer, F. E. (1990). Prospective study of estrogen replacement therapy and risk of breast cancer in postmenopausal women. *J. Am. Med. Assoc.*, **264**, 2648–53

48. Anderson, T., Battersby, S., King, R., McPherson, K. and Going, J. (1989). Oral contraceptive use influences resting breast proliferation. *Hum. Pathol.*, **20**, 1139–44

49. Boston Collaborative Drug Surveillance Program (1974). Surgically confirmed gall-bladder disease, venous thromboembolism and breast tumors in relation to post-menopausal estrogen therapy. *N. Engl. J. Med.*, **290**, 15–19

50. Campbell, S. and Whitehead, M. I. (1982). Potency and hepatocellular effects of oestrogens. In Van Keep, P. A., Utian, W. H. and Vermuelen, A. (eds.) *The Controversial Climacteric*, pp. 103–25. (Lancaster: MTP Press)

51. Lievertz, R. W. (1987). Pharmacology and pharmacokinetics of estrogens. *Am. J. Obstet. Gynecol.*, **156**, 1289–93

52. Cope, E. (1976). Physical changes associated with the post-menopausal years. In Campbell, S. (ed.) *The Manage-ment of the Menopause and Postmenopausal Years*, p. 33. (Lancaster: MTP Press)

53. Population Projections Series PP2 No. 16. Office of Population Census and Surveys

54. Speroff, L., Glass, R. and Case, N. (1983). *Clinical Gynecological Endocrinology and Infertility*. (Baltimore: Williams and Wilkins)

55. Whitehead, M. and Studd, J. W. W. (1988). Selection of patients for treatment. Which therapy and for how long? In Studd, J. W. W. and Whitehead, M. I. (eds.) *The Menopause*, p. 117. (Oxford: Blackwell Scientific)

56. Molnar, G. W. (1975). Body temperatures during menopausal hot flushes. *J. Appl. Physiol.*, **38**, 499–503

57. Dempster, D., Shane, E., Horbert, W. and Lindsay, R. (1986). A simple method for correlative scanning electron microscopy of human iliac crest biopsies. *Am. J. Bone Min. Res.*, **1**, 15–21

58. 1983–85, Hospital In-Patient Enquiry: 1988 onwards. *Hospital Episode Statistics*

59. Colditz, G. A., Willett, W. C., Stampfer, M. J., Rosner, B., Speizer, F. E. and Hennekens, C. H. (1987). Menopause and the risk of coronary heart disease in women. *N. Engl. J. Med.*, **316**, 1105–10

60. Stevenson, J. C., Crook, D. and Godsland, I. F. (1993). Influence of age and menopause on serum lipids and lipoproteins in healthy women. *Atherosclerosis*, **98**, 83–90

61. Mortality statistics: cause. Series DH2 no. 14. Office of Population Census and Surveys

62. Hospital In-Patient Enquiry Series MB4 no. 29

63. Gambrell, R. D. Jr. (1983). Breast disease in the post-menopausal years. *Sem. Reprod. Endocrinol.*, **1**, 27–40

64. Key, T. J. and Pike, M. C. (1988). The role of oestrogens and progestogens in the epidemiology and prevention of breast carcinoma. *Eur. J. Cancer Clin. Oncol.*, **24**, 29–43

65. Mashchak, C. A., Lobo, R. A., Dozono-Takano, R., Eggena, P., Nakamura, R. M., Brenner, P. F. and Mischell, D. R. (1982). Comparison of pharmacodynamic properties of various estrogen formulations. *Am. J. Obstet. Gynecol.*, **144**, 511–18

66. Barlow, D. H., Abdullah, H. I., Roberts, A. D., Al-Azzawi, F., Leggate, I. and Hart, D. M. (1986). Long-term hormone

implant therapy – hormonal and clinical effects. *Obstet. Gynecol.*, **67**, 321–5

67. Whitehead, M. and Godfree, V. (1992). *Hormone Replacement Therapy: Your Questions Answered*, p. 99. (Edinburgh: Churchill Livingstone)

68. Jensen, J. and Christiansen, C. (1983). Dose response and withdrawal effects of climacteric symptoms after hormonal replacement therapy. A placebo-controlled therapeutic trial. *Maturitas*, **5**, 125–33

69. Campbell, S. and Whitehead, M. I. (1977). Oestrogen therapy and the menopausal syndrome. In Greenblatt, R. B. and Studd, J. W. W. (eds.) *Clinics in Obstetrics and Gynecology*, Vol. 4, no. 1, pp. 31–47. (Philadelphia: W. B. Saunders)

70. Padwick, M. L., Endacott, J. and Whitehead, M. I. (1985). Efficacy, acceptability and metabolic effects of transdermal estradiol in the management of postmenopasual women. *Am. J. Obstet. Gynecol.*, **152**, 1085–91

71. Schiff, I., Tulchinsky, D. and Ryan, K. J. (1977). Vaginal absorption of oestrone and oestradiol 17-β. *Fertil. Steril.*, **28**, 1063

72. Dyer, G. I., Young, O., Townsend, P. T., Collins, W. P. and Whitehead, M. I. (1982). Dose-related changes in vaginal cytology after topical conjugated equine oestrogens. *Br. Med. J.*, **284**, 789

73. Cardozo, L. D., Gibb, D. M. F., Studd, J. W. W., Tuck, S. M., Thom, M. H. and Cooper, D. J. (1983). The effects of subcutaneous hormone implant during the climacteric. *Maturitas*, **5**, 177–84

74. Brincat, M., Studd, J., O'Dowd, T., Magos, A., Cardozo, L. D., Wardle, P. J. and Cooper, D. (1984). Subcutaneous hormone implants for the control of climacteric symptoms. *Lancet*, **1**, 16–18

75. Fraser, D., Padwick, M. L., Whitehead, M. I., Coffer, A. and King, R., J. B. (1991). Presence of an oestradiol receptor-related protein in the skin: changes during the normal menstrual cycle. *Br. J. Obstet. Gynaecol.*, **98**, 1277–82

76. Melton, J., Wahner, H., Richelson, L., O'Fallon, M. and Riggs, B. (1986). Osteoporosis and the risk of hip fracture. *Am. J. Epidemiol.*, **124**, 254–61

77. Quigley, M., Purvis, L., Martin, M., Burnier, A. and Brooks, P. (1987). Estrogen therapy arrests bone loss in elderly women. *Am. J. Obstet. Gynecol.*, **156**, 1516–21

78. Lindsay, R. and Tohme, J. (1990). Estrogen treatment of patients with established postmenopausal osteoporosis. *Obstet. Gynecol.*, **76**, 290–5

79. Stevenson, J. C., Cust, M., Gangar, K. F., Hillard, T. C., Lees, B. and Whitehead, M. I. (1990). Effects of transdermal versus oral hormone replacement therapy on bone density in the spine and proximal femur of postmenopausal women. *Lancet*, **335**, 265–9

80. Studd, J., Savvas, M., Watson, N., Garnett, T., Fogelman, I. and Cooper, D. (1990). The relationship between plasma oestradiol and the increase in bone density in the postmenopausal women after treatment with subcutaneous implants. *Am. J. Obstet. Gynecol.*, **163**, 474–9

81. Stampfer, M. J., Willett, W. C., Colditz, G. A., Rosner, B., Speizer, F. E. and Hennekens, C. H. (1985). A prospective study of postmenopausal estrogen therapy and coronary heart disease. *N. Engl. J. Med.*, **313**, 1044–9

82. Henderson, B. E., Ross, R. K., Paganini-Hill, A. and Mack, T. M. (1986). Estrogen use and cardiovascular disease. *Am. J. Obstet. Gynecol.*, **154**, 1181–6

83. Gruchow, H. W., Anderson, A. J., Barboriak, J. J. and Sobocinski, K. A. (1988). Postmenopausal use of estrogen and occlusion of coronary arteries. *Am. Heart J.*, **115**, 954–63

84. Sullivan, J. M., Van der Zwaag, R., Hughes, J. P., Maddock, V., Kroetz, F. W., Ramanathan, K. B. and Mirvis, D. M. (1990). Estrogen replacement and coronary artery disease – effect on survival in postmenopausal women. *Arch. Intern. Med.*, **150**, 2557–62

85. Ottoson, U. B., Johansson, B. G. and von Schoultz, B. (1985). Subfractions of high-density lipoprotein cholesterol during estrogen replacement therapy: a comparison between progestogens and natural progesterone. *Am. J. Obstet. Gynecol.*, **151**, 746–50

86. Hillard, T. C., Bourne, T. H., Whitehead, M. I., Crayford, T. B., Collins, W. P. and Campbell, S. (1992). Differential effects of transdermal estradiol and sequential progestogens on impedance to flow within the uterine arteries of postmenopausal women. *Fertil. Steril.*, **58**, 959–63

87. Whitehead, M. I., Hillard, T. C. and Crook, D. (1990). The role and use of progestogens. *Obstet. Gynecol.*, **75**, 59–76S

88. Lane, G., Siddle, N. C., Ryder, T. A., Pryse-Davies, J., King, R. J. B. and Whitehead, M. I. (1983). Dose dependent effects of oral progesterone on the oestrogenised postmenopausal endometrium. *Br. Med. J.*, **287**, 1241–5

89. Whitehead, M. I., Townsend, P. T., Pryse-Davies, J. Ryder, T., Lane, G., Siddle, N. C. and King, R. J. B. (1982). Effects of various types and dosages of progestogens on the postmenopausal endometrium. *J. Reprod. Med.*, **27**, 539–48

90. Nomura, A. M. Y., Kolonel, L. N., Hirohata, T. and Lee, J. (1986). The association of replacement estrogens with breast cancer. *Int. J. Cancer*, **37**, 49–53

91. Buring, J. E., Hennekens, C. H., Lipnick, R. J., Willett, W., Stampfer, M. J., Rosner, B., Peto, R. and Speizer, F. E. (1987). A prospective cohort study of postmenopausal hormone use and risk of breast cancer in US women. *Am. J. Epidemiol.*, **125**, 939–47

92. Mills, P. K., Beeson, W. L., Phillips, R. L. and Fraser, G. E. (1989). Prospective study of exogenous hormone use and breast cancer in Seventh-day Adventists. *Cancer*, **64**, 591–7

93. Sherman, B., Wallace, R. and Beau, J. (1983). Estrogen use and breast cancer. Interaction with body mass. *Cancer*, **51**, 1527–31

94. McDonald, J. A., Weiss, N. S., Daling, J. R., Francis, A. M. and Poliss, A. R. L. (1986). Menopausal estrogen use and the risk of breast cancer. *Breast Cancer Res. Treatm.*, **7**, 193–9

95. Hulka, B., Chambless, L., Dubner, D. and Wilkinson, W. (1982). Breast cancer and estrogen replacement therapy. *Am. J. Obstet. Gynecol.*, **143**, 638–44

96. Bergkvist, L., Adami, H. -O., Persson, I., Hoover, R. and Chairer, K. (1989). Risk of breast cancer after estrogen and progestin replacement. *N. Engl. J. Med.*, **321**, 293–7

Index